Praise for Mark Whitwell and
The Promise of Love, Sex, and Intimacy

"In his book, Mark shares the importance of breathing to energize ourselves. Breathe and let go. Read this book."

—Deepak Chopra

"An incredible business tool that has given me financial, emotional, and spiritual freedom. [Your Seven-Minute Wonder] will give you the feeling of intimacy with life and one's principal relationships."

—Rinaldo S. Brutoco, founding president & CEO, World Business Academy

"I have prescribed Mark's seven-minute breathing and movement routine to hundreds of my patients, who have reported a renaissance of energy in their lives, while experiencing deeper sleep, a stronger body composition, more vitality, less depression, and an astonishingly improved sensuality and sex drive."

—Prudence Hall, MD, founder, Hall Center Venice

"Mark offers us a simple, self-respecting practice that gives astounding results. To trust breath as the source of life gives powerful intimacy to self and others."

—Jackie Mills, group fitness director, Les Mills International

"A great gift. I do it every day. It's the perfect way to begin anew—bringing everyone to a beautiful beginning with each day, each breath, closer to God, to source, to life."

—Richard Baskin, executive director,
Urban Zen Integrative Therapy Programs

"Mark helps us to realize genuine love, sex, and intimacy with Your Seven-Minute Wonder. *The Promise of Love, Sex, and Intimacy* helps us to have an intimate connection to what this precious life has to offer, and practicing it can *transform your life from inside out.*"

—Kiyoshi Suzaki, author of *Results from the Heart*,
foreword by the Dalai Lama

The Promise
of
Love, Sex, and Intimacy

How a Simple Breathing Practice

Will Enrich Your Life Forever

MARK WHITWELL

ATRIA BOOKS

NEW YORK   LONDON   TORONTO   SYDNEY   NEW DELHI

ATRIA BOOKS

A Division of Simon & Schuster, Inc.
1230 Avenue of the Americas
New York, NY 10020

First Atria Books hardcover edition June 2012

ATRIA B O O K S and colophon are trademarks of Simon & Schuster, Inc.

For information about special discounts for bulk purchases, please contact Simon & Schuster Special Sales at 1-866-506-1949 or business@simonandschuster.com.

The Simon & Schuster Speakers Bureau can bring authors to your live event. For more information or to book an event, contact the Simon & Schuster Speakers Bureau at 1-866-248-3049 or visit our website at www.simonspeakers.com.

Designed by Kyoko Watanabe

Manufactured in the United States of America

10   9   8   7   6   5   4   3   2   1

Library of Congress Cataloging-in-Publication Data

Whitwell, Mark.
  The promise of love, sex and intimacy : how a simple breathing practice will enrich your life forever / by Mark Whitwell.
     p. cm.
1. Breathing exercises. 2. Respiration—Religious aspects. 3. Intimacy (Psychology) 4. Love. I. Title.
  RA782.W45 2012
  613'.192—dc23

                                                                  2012014888

ISBN 978-1-4516-4988-8
ISBN 978-1-4516-4989-5 (ebook)

I dedicate this book to you! You are holding in your hands and heart the promise that delivers everything you ever needed. You are the extreme intelligence, beauty, and function of Life. You are at One with Life, yet an utterly unique appearance of Life. Nature does not work in models, only "one-offs," and there is no one remotely like you in the universe. Your Life is operating in an extraordinary way. No one need give you this intelligence and no one can take it from you. I therefore offer you nothing except the practical means by which you can participate in your own Wonder day by day. This is my promise to you. I dedicate this work to everyOne and offer the realistic practice, which fulfills all inspirations. And to all those who will pass it on until we all get it. Like my friend Peter Occhiogrosso, our midwife of the Promise all the way. When Peter first taught the Promise Practice at a United Nations conference, addressing a multicultural audience that included many diverse national, ethnic, class, religious, and nonreligious points of view, he discovered how easy it was to give the gift and how wholly helpful it was to every person gathered there.

Contents

PART II:

Your Seven-Minute Wonder!

Foreword

HERE IS A SIMPLE, IRREFUTABLE TRUTH: WE BREATHE. We all have that in common. We breathe, and we all do it the same way, basically. Air is inhaled when the diaphragm and intercostal muscles enlarge the chest, and air is exhaled when these muscles relax.

Rich, poor, fat, skinny, black, white, male, female, gay, straight, old, young, enemy, or friend—we breathe. We are united in breath, and we all do it so well that it keeps us alive and active for years. Even if your breathing is impaired, it hasn't stopped. Something is breathing you. Some power. Something you can rely on. What a gift! And it arrives fully assembled. Already perfected.

What if the same could be said about other aspects of our lives? It may be possible that we're more okay than we think. Here you are, here I am, beautifully realized and wonderfully acceptable just as we are. I can't speak for you, but I just felt a wave of relief.

This relief is what our breath provides moment by moment. With each breath, you don't seek or strive for some better way to exist, or a more loving relationship, or more rewarding work. There is no faraway version of yourself. You're right here, right now.

That's the message of the book you're holding in your hands. It's more of a reminder than a message. Our relationship to our breath, and to our lives, is intimate and present. When we remember this, many stresses and struggles fall away.

And there is a way to remember; a practical way that can be applied for a few minutes every day. Breathe in and raise your arms. Breathe out and lower them again. The intimacy of breath and movement will spread into your life and into the lives of others. This is the promise being made here.

Myself, I speak with no special authority. I'm not a meditator or a spiritual seeker or a health expert. I'm a Los Angeles screenwriter and movie director, a father of two grown children, a tax-paying consumer, and an unambitious ukulele player.

Yet I'm writing the foreword to this book because three years ago I took up the practice that is being offered here, and I can tell you with certainty that *it has changed my life*!

Strike that. It has relieved me of the nerve-wracking *struggle* to change my life. To scramble after some impossible image of myself. To put on pause the Here and Now of life, while reaching for something unreachable. That was me for decades: straining to get ahead in my work, desiring women who couldn't possibly exist, dreaming of success, or wealth, or heaven, and missing out, very often, on the beautiful reality of earth. Missing out on intimacy, with myself and with others. Too busy to stop—and catch my breath.

I now start my day by moving and breathing without

any agenda except to move and breathe. For a few minutes, that's all. As simple as that sounds, those few minutes have awakened an intrinsic intimacy, with myself and with others, that enriches the rest of my day.

And here's the irony and the bonus: my work has become fulfilling and productive, my health and physical fitness have improved, and all my relationships have deepened and sweetened and bloomed.

Stop looking and start living. That's the essence—the heart and soul—of the Promise and of Mark Whitwell's teaching. And it comes with a practical method that anyone who breathes can apply.

Try it. You won't become enlightened or superhuman or turn into something you never were—and that's the best news of all. You'll befriend the human being you've always been: the walking, talking, laughing, breathing miracle that is *you*.

Bob Dolman
Venice, California, 2012

Introduction

What you truly need is not secret knowledge but a realistic practice that will allow you to navigate through the noise and chaos of your life, and direct you to the Source of peace and power that is in you.

WE MIGHT HAVE THE FASTEST AND HOTTEST SMARTphones, age-defying beauty treatments, or a plethora of pills to deal with the chaos of our modern lives. We might follow a most sincere religious or spiritual path, or we might take an atheistic or agnostic position in life. But in the midst of this busy world, we have lost touch with the gentle truth that is the unseen guide within us all. What we really need is something more potent and direct: love, intimacy, and sex.

When we are well loved, we inevitably give love to those around us. It is like having enough food or enough money to meet all your needs; you just naturally want to share. When we lack, however, we withdraw and seek answers in all the wrong places. Instead of prioritizing love, sex, and intimacy, many of us succumb to social pressures that encourage us to be sexier, richer, prettier, smarter.

We buy into the idea that our happiness will result from getting that dream body, house, lover, family, job, bank account, and on and on. Surely everything would be perfect then, right?

In this competitive culture, it's hard to resist these ideals and expectations.

By struggling to live up to them, many of us find ourselves stressed out, overworked, in debt, dealing with strained relationships, or searching in vain for a partner. Somewhere along the line, the formula for "success" and "happiness" has gone awry and is taking us further away from what will actually soothe us.

For many, the new age movement has offered alternative solutions to this growing dissatisfaction with materialistic lifestyles. Yet this too can encourage us to strive for impossible ideals. A spiritual path implies that we are not there yet. By seeking some kind of "enlightenment," you may lose sight of the fact that you have everything you need right in front of you. You already are a living, breathing, perfect expression of life. You don't need to attain it—you *are* it!

Ironically, spiritual seeking clouds our ability to see this truth. There is no such thing as enlightenment. It's a concept that has been made up and imposed upon us by the charm and persuasion of so-called spiritual authorities. There is only life itself, reality itself, that beats the heart and moves the breath and sex. So stop trying to "be here now"—you *are* here now! The power, intelligence, beauty, and wonder of life are already given.

Happiness arises when you relax into the reality of

your natural condition. This intimate participation in your own life is the greatest gift you can give yourself and everyone around you, and the best model that you can offer your children and your community.

The Promise will help you see this profound truth. More important, it will give you the practical means to experience it. That is my intention in writing this book. It is a practical, sincere guide to living, the self-help book to end all self-help books. The practice offered in these pages is derived from timeless wisdom that provides not only the essential knowledge but also the practical steps to implement your real needs and desires. Here is the practicum, the all-purpose "how-to" manual for everything that has ever inspired you or will inspire you. *In*-spire, breathe in. It is a soft message for hard times.

A Quick Overview

The first section of the book will provide you with the philosophical basis of this practice, outlining why intimacy is as close and as necessary as your breath is to your body. It explores how we have become disconnected from the extreme intelligence that is life, and the impact that institutional religion, new age philosophies, and pop culture have had on our sense of self and our ability to relate to others in powerful ways. These same influences have perpetuated negative and exaggerated ideas about sexuality. This section will help you examine your sexuality and beliefs, and consider to what extent these beliefs are positive, empowering, and supportive. You deserve your life to be intimate, powerful, and full of love. This is wholly within your grasp.

The second half of this book, "Your Seven-Minute Wonder!," presents a few simple exercises of synchronized breath and movement. This brief and very enjoyable practice will allow you to experience an exquisite connection with the source of life and all of life's relationships, felt through breath, movement, and sex. It will nurture you, regenerate you, and heal you.

The Promise is my commitment to you and my belief in the power that I know these practices hold. By bringing this practice into your life, you are beginning a process that will not only provide immediate benefits but will also leave you with rewards, seen and unseen, that are ongoing and cumulative.

To be effective, the practice requires the energy and commitment of two parties: you and I. I ask you to promise to start practicing Your Seven-Minute Wonder, naturally and not obsessively, as part of your daily routine. Whether it is in the morning or the evening, allow yourself no less than seven minutes to establish this practice, and sustain it for forty days. You may begin anytime while reading this book; please feel free to move through the different sections as it suits you.

In return for your promise, I promise that you will come to embody the power that lives and breathes you. You will experience the reality of life that expresses itself in you, *as* you, as well as a deep sense of authenticity in all areas, including love, sex, health, cultural participation, or religious inspiration. What is unimportant will naturally fall away, and you will feel yourself step into your power with quiet grace and certainty. Through the medium of your body and breath, intimacy will ripple throughout your life and relationships in beautiful and exciting ways.

I promise.

Mark Whitwell
Los Angeles, 2012

PART I

A Promise That Delivers

CHAPTER 1

What Is the Promise?

*Life is not a desperate, fearful affair of struggle, ill
health, and death. Life is an eternal flow of nurturing
that cannot be lost. You do not even have to search for
it, because it is utterly given. You are loved and cared
for completely.*

ONE NIGHT ABOUT FORTY YEARS AGO, I WAS STANDING
on a rooftop in a country thousands of miles from my
home in the South Pacific, when I suddenly experienced
a sense of wonder. It was sublime: a deep, spontaneous
feeling of well-being, of bliss, of love. I felt completely
nurtured, my whole body fully integrated with everything
in the natural world and with everyOne around me.

What had caused this wonder-full feeling? There was
no external reason: no girl, no drugs, no hit on the head
with a peacock feather from Swami Knowitallananda. Yet
there I was, under a full moon and infinite stars, blissfully
alive and certain of the simplest realization.

"This body loves its breath," I whispered to the night
crickets.

Like a man loves God, like a woman loves a man, like a bee loves nectar. "This exhalation completely loves the inhalation," I said aloud. "And it's so easy!"

I'd traveled a great many miles, looking for answers outside of myself, before coming to this realization. Having lived through the usual troubles of a Western teenager, growing up in New Zealand and attending a church-run school, I knew that there had to be something better than what society was dishing up at the time. Our parents had won the last world war and given us free speech and a free life, for which I was profoundly grateful. But I couldn't shake the feeling in my bones that there had to be more than the commercialism I saw around me, and the academic system that was merely preparing us for the universities. And so I took off around the world in search of wisdom—or something—among the great traditions that I'd heard and read about.

Landing on the subcontinent of South Asia, I sought out the masters of the ancient traditions. There was no Internet back then, and no books had yet been published about their teachings, so I had to conduct my search by a combination of intuition and trial and error. The first thing I discovered was that "spiritual life" was a major industry there. The wisdom teachings that I was seeking were available, in most instances, for a price. "That's all right," I thought, "everyone needs to earn a living." But I found out over time that doing business was more important to most of these "holy men" than the well-being of the people who came to them for teaching—not only Westerners but also the local seekers.

Among the shoddy spiritual goods being sold in the marketplace, I found little that was useful. I had to sift through a ton of sand before I located any jewels. But the painstaking search was worth it. I was able to find a handful of teachers who were as appalled by these spiritual hucksters as I was.

The foremost among these men became my friend as well as my teacher. Indeed, he told me that the true teacher is "no more than a friend and no less than a friend." In the end, there was no need for a teaching at all, he said, because the universe knows exactly what it is doing with each and every person.

"I have nothing to teach," this extraordinary man said to me. "I have no message for mankind."

"Now, *there's* a teaching!" I thought.

"The whole world has been seduced by enlightenment," this man said.

In a single stroke, he undermined the spell—the hoax—that my search for wisdom had cast over me. I'd been determined to know what was *really* going on, what worked and what did not. What was the key? What was the essential information that I needed—and that the world needed? I had been seduced by the idea that you could attain permanent happiness, and that's what I was looking for: in a word, enlightenment! Now this man was telling me with authority that looking for enlightenment was itself the problem, because it implied that I didn't already have it.

"Stop looking and start living," he told me. "The whole idea of trying to *become* something is a denial of who you are."

Having said that, he showed me a physical practice that he followed every day. He also mentioned a word that I had previously associated with a series of acrobatic postures that you do on a rubber mat while wearing a leotard or a loincloth. But I instinctively knew that he wasn't talking about some system of aggressive exercise for weight loss! His practice consisted of simply participating in the movement of Source Reality through his body and breath. (By Source Reality I mean the power of the universe that moves everything.) It wasn't about some abstract concept of enlightenment. It was about discovering the natural intimacy of body, breath, and movement. He would move and breathe on the floor with me to show how to participate in life instead of attempting to manipulate life with physical contortions or meditation, like spiritual gymnastics. He would laugh and gossip about the ordinary delights of life, and was always helpful in the most practical ways.

He demonstrated his practice with no sense of effort or strain. Watching him, I realized that the forcible teaching of postures and meditation that I had encountered elsewhere is an imposition on the human system. He was emphatic that most teachers were just in it for the business. Since I had already begun to sense that, I was drawn to his "nonteaching." This man was so adamant that truth could not be bought or sold. Truth did not belong to anyone in particular or, in other words, it belonged to everyOne and every thing. It could not be found, because you never lose it—and the very act of looking for it implies its absence. Whereas truth really is intrinsic, and always present in your innate, natural state.

So it's the act of looking for it that is the problem. All we need do in life is to participate in it. To emphasize this point, he would say bluntly, "Don't turn my words into a teaching, or me into one of those teachers exploiting the gullibility of the people to look for something they have never lost." He would refuse to allow people to copyright his words in books so they could be used to make money and exploit people. Sometimes I expressed my wonder at something especially mind blowing that he had said, adding that I wanted to let the world know what he was teaching me. But he used to joke, "Don't tell people I said these things. Tell them you said it, and you'll make a lot of money." He would also say things like, "To be yourself requires extraordinary intelligence. You are blessed with that intelligence; nobody need give it to you, nobody can take it away from you."

After having wasted my time, my money, and not a little of my faith in humankind, I had finally found a spiritual master I could believe in.

"Now," this man said, "life begins."

I began at once to make this practice an essential part of my daily routine. It wasn't difficult to do; it required very little time or effort. In about twenty minutes, I'd been taught how to link my breath to my whole body movement. At first I wasn't sure if I was doing it right or if there were any real benefits to be gained. I wasn't getting a sweaty workout, my heart wasn't pounding, my muscles weren't pumped or strained. Yet by doing this easy practice every day, naturally and not obsessively, I gradually experienced something that I had never been conscious of before:

My body and my breath were connected—intimately.

That intimacy fully awakened as I stood on that rooftop, in love with life under a full moon. My teacher (I considered him a teacher, even if he did not) had passed on to me the primal wisdom of the ancient world—a physical practice that had almost been lost and forgotten. It was a lifeline, I realized, that linked me not only to my inner self but also to the outside world. Intimacy between the body and its breath tangibly reveals every kind of intimacy with the natural state, including the absolute Source that sustains and nurtures all creation.

The next day I asked my teacher about my rooftop insight. "I think I've discovered the secret," I said. "It is the breath moving in the whole body. It is the whole body participating in the breath."

"Yes," he said. "But I wanted you to discover this yourself, not just tell it to you like another abstract fact to learn."

By writing this book, I am passing on this ancient practice to you, and I want *you* to discover it for yourself the same way that I did.

By doing it.

By making a Promise to yourself: to do a daily practice that I call Your Seven-Minute Wonder. For that is all that's required to enrich the intimacy in your life: a minimum of seven minutes every day.

Coming Down from the Mountain: Giving It All Away

The Promise that you hold in your hands is truly giving it all away. I'm not holding on to information but giving to you now what I've learned with others. Having spent years learning their wisdom, I then spent many more years extracting and refining the core of it in a way that Westerners—and other Easterners, for that matter—could easily apply to their daily lives. Back in New Zealand, I had been a college teacher, and my father a dedicated professor of history, so I knew I had within me the capacity to learn and to pass on what I'd learned to others. Later I became a telecommunications guru and an information technology consultant, suddenly aware that we now had the capability of spreading this jewel of intimate human wisdom to the entire world. We could, at the speed of light, pass it on to everyOne to be nurtured—starting today.

The Promise I offer you in this book is the missing link. It is the distillation of the ancient wisdom of the body that I learned from my teachers. It represents the practical means that allow you to realize the sublimity of your inspiration and all your desires. This truth was always there in the founding of doctrine but lay forgotten within the twists and turns and power struggles of abstract belief systems.

Yet what exactly *is* the truth that I discovered? *That intimacy with all ordinary conditions reveals the Source of all conditions, because the Source and the "seen" are one.* This is the grand announcement of all traditions. In simpler terms: the Creator and creation really are One. What you see all around you and what you experience inside you are identical with the Source of all life. There is no difference. That being true, then it follows that intimacy with the ordinary is full and sufficient, and reveals all that we need to know. The realization of this—and the *practice* of it—is what I mean by the Promise.

The Promise is not religion. It is a practical means for realizing the Source of all truth. I am back from the mountain, back from my meetings with the hidden masters, and have found a way to synthesize what they gave me to give to you in this pithy, easily understood formula. *It simply works.*

Take the pill, and you will feel great. It's logical, even mathematical: $2 + 2 = 4$. We had caring teachers at school who insisted that we know our math, that we be able to read and write and think—dear friends who would never let us out of school without that precious knowledge. But they never told us what we actually need most of all. No one had ever given them this gift for a hard time so that they could pass it on to us.

Yet I am about to tell you. It will help you in all your endeavors, and it is universal to all cultures, nationalities, faiths, lifestyles, and people everywhere. And it's no exaggeration. If you promise me to practice these easy breath and body movements for seven minutes a day, I promise you a wonder-full result that will be a catalyst for you to enjoy your wildest dreams. Love, bliss, sex, and intimacies of every kind will be realized, including the mystery source of civilization and the abundance of all life.

Why Seven Minutes?

The practice that I am asking you to do is called Your Seven-Minute Wonder. It is a physical practice that is pleasurable and invigorating, and if you choose to extend it beyond seven minutes, please do. But commit to at least seven minutes. It's the minimum amount of time you'll need in order to enjoy the many benefits described in this book.

I came up with Your Seven-Minute Wonder by simple trial and error. I used to encourage my friends to do *twenty* minutes of moving and breathing practice daily, and they never would! Or they would for a while and give up. Some would do an hour obsessively as a novelty, but when the novelty wore off, they also gave up.

I whittled it down to fifteen minutes. This still didn't work. Down to ten minutes. They were *still* too busy—or so they said. Then one day, sitting outside the Sydney Opera House, I asked a friend at a conference, "Would you do this practice for *seven* minutes each day?"

There was a long, pregnant pause. The world seemed to stop. I could see in my friend's face that she was thinking about those seven minutes, and that she couldn't find a reason to refuse them.

I waited, and finally she said, with an easy smile, "That's doable! I will. I promise."

The sky grew golden, there was a crack of thunder and a lightning bolt, and the universe appeared to open up—or at least that's how excited I became. I knew in that moment that seven minutes was the right amount of time to ask of people. My friend there in Sydney was my evidence: she was *happy* to practice for seven minutes a day. She could easily fit it into her full and busy life.

And she did! She made a promise to herself that she could keep.

That very week, I created the iPhone app called iPromise! Here was Your Seven-Minute Wonder in the palm of your hand. I also began at once to teach Your Seven-Minute Wonder in classes and workshops. My students readily made the Promise, as if seven minutes were the magic number. And those who kept their Promise (I'm pleased to report that most people do) have experienced many positive results.

Some of those experiences have been included throughout this book, and the practice itself, Your Seven-Minute Wonder, which I also refer to as "the Promise Practice," is described with simple instructions in the second half of the book. On pages 265–268 I've also included video links describing the steps of the practice. You're welcome to jump ahead and learn the practice now if you'd like. In fact, I recommend it. It will enrich your reading experience if you do.

Seven minutes a day. And if you keep it up for at least forty days, I promise you this: you will establish a positive, permanent habit that will enrich your life, and the lives of everyone around you.

CHAPTER 2

Inhaling Intimacy

To the ancient masters, a powerful physical practice was not merely a form of exercise meant to increase flexibility or fitness. It was a spiritual way of life based on the intuitive understanding that everything is arising continuously from one Nurturing Source.

HOW CLOSE IS YOUR BREATH TO YOUR BODY? HOW much do your breath and body need each other? Try not breathing for a few minutes, and you'll find out just how much!

Your body loves its breath. And yet breathing isn't as simple as it might seem. For many of us, the inhalation is qualitatively different from the exhalation. Most of the time, we take short, narrow breaths that don't calm and refresh our body, or engage the male and female aspects of the body and psyche that coexist within each of us. Muscle-bound men, for instance, can exhale well enough because that's about strength. But they can't *inhale* very well. Inhaling requires receptivity, and often the strongest people have difficulty being receptive.

Bill's Story: Waiting to Inhale

One time in New Zealand, I was working with a police-man named Bill, who couldn't inhale very well because he was so strong and trying too hard: he had become muscle-bound. True to form, Bill was making a muscular effort to breathe as I instructed him, conscientiously sucking air through his nostrils, but he wasn't participating in his inhalation. Even moving his arms in rhythm to the breath didn't help, as it does for many people.

I taught Bill how to breathe so that the breath goes through the nostrils but isn't drawn in by them. Instead the larynx, or voice box, becomes the controlling center of the breath, and the air goes straight into the upper chest and rib cage. This is the same breath that your body normally uses when you fall asleep—but, of course, you're not aware of it, because by then you're unconscious. Sometimes, though, you can perceive that beautiful moment when the body catches its sweet, deep, refreshing, whole body breath as you plunge into an energizing sleep. Or, if you listen to your partner sleeping, you'll hear what I mean. You can also think of it as Darth Vader breathing, because it sounds like a soft version of the breath of that guy from *Star Wars*!

Once I got Bill to breathe this way, which took him only a minute or two to master, I asked him to duplicate the sound of his exhale on the inhale. This was another way to balance the polarities within him—matching the strong, masculine exhalation with the receptive, feminine inhalation. That's the key to the principle of what I call "strength receiving": the ability to engage both the male and female aspects that we all have within us, whatever our gender and whatever our sexual orientation.

That took a little longer, but Bill got it soon enough. A smile lit up his face as he realized that something that had sounded impossible or esoteric was within his grasp. Then I could start exploring movement in coordination with his breathing.

Breathing Practice

Later in the book, I'll discuss in more detail the technique that I taught Bill, when I show you how to do Your Seven-Minute Wonder. On pages 265–268 I've also included video tags that describe the Promise Practice. But you can try this right now if you'd like to get a sense of where we'll be going.

Begin by taking a few breaths in a relaxed standing or seated position. If you're sitting in a chair, try sitting toward the front with your spine straight and your feet flat on the floor. Keeping the mouth closed softly, breathe in and out through the nose. The aim is not to use the nostrils as if you are sniffing but to regulate the flow of the breath at the back of the throat. Begin to whisper a soft *haaaaa* sound with your mouth open, making the sound on both inhalation and exhalation. After you have practiced this a few times, close your mouth and see if you can produce a similar sound and sensation while keeping the nostrils passive. You can also try humming with your mouth closed. Keep breathing that way but stop making an audible hum. You will feel the air in the nostrils very lightly, but the suction of the throat is what regulates the airflow.

It may come easily or take a few attempts to master, but with practice and persistence, it will evolve from something that may feel slightly strained and unnatural to something that seems instinctual and pleasurable. There are many advantages to directing the breath in this manner. First, making the breath audible provides you with a point on which to focus. Accept the fact that your mind will wander from time to time during any practice. Through careful attention to the breath, you provide yourself with a clear and tangible "point of return" that you can use throughout the various stages of practice.

More than anything, though, this kind of breathing makes it easier to breathe deeply and evenly, without great effort. In a way, it's teaching you to be more receptive; to be aware of your breath without straining to suck a lot of air into your lungs. Once you're able to breathe in this way, controlling your breath with the larynx instead of the nostrils, you'll start to hear and feel the difference from your accustomed way of breathing. Try doing this for a few moments several times a day, just for the enjoyment of feeling and hearing your breath. You'll see what I mean by *loving your breath*. Begin when you're alone and in a calm situation, then branch out. You can try it while walking or driving, or when you're with a group of people at a store or in a meeting. (You can modify the volume so that it's virtually inaudible to anyone but you.) You can even use it in any mildly stressful situation that arises. Instead of dissociating yourself from what's happening—"witnessing," as some teachers of "awareness," or "insight," meditation advise—you'll get a sense of being grounded, calmer, receptive, and better able to deal with the situation. You'll be more intimately connected to yourself and to those around you. You are "with" your experience. You embrace your relatedness. You do not exist to be the mere observer of whatever is happening but to be at one with your life and all arising conditions.

We'll make extended use of this kind of breathing later on, but this way you can get a head start while enjoying the sensation of using your breath in a whole new way. Be sure to pay attention to any resistance you may feel in teaching yourself this practice. We are socially conditioned to achieve; to be successful by acquiring things (*grasping* might be a better word). We're taught to be strong, yet we have trouble receiving freely. By freeing yourself to open the front of your chest to receive the breath in this way, you become more receptive to your own experience of life. Combined with the simple movement I'll be showing you, this will also make you more receptive to other people.

When I spoke later to Bill the policeman, he told me excitedly that he had learned to receive. He was so surprised to find what it had done for him and his wife. I knew that without having the practical means, Bill would not enjoy any improvement in his intimate relationship. He had admitted to his previous life habit of trying to control his circumstances only, and had become unreceptive to his wife's needs in a number of ways. He reported that he felt the most relaxed and peaceful ever. It was a strangely familiar yet forgotten feeling that connected him to his youth, when he would run carefree in the fields. Later Bill would tell me that his Seven-Minute Wonder was the best thing he had ever done for himself and his family, and he was enjoying his life and wife in a brand-new way.

That's how the practice can improve the level of sexual intimacy you allow into your life. One reason why people often feel guilty about their sexuality is that they tend to think of sex as some instinctive act of pleasure seeking. It *is* that on one level, just as eating or playing are—and we don't normally feel guilty about *those* activities. But the deepest joy of lovemaking comes from opening up and being receptive to another person. When the nerve endings in the front of your body uncurl, like the petals of a flower opening to a honeybee, this has a profound effect on how you relate to others, whether as friends, colleagues, or intimate sexual partners.

Strength Receiving

Lack of receptiveness can play out in other areas of our life and health as well. When you've been brought up from early childhood to be strong and to achieve, but haven't learned receptivity, then by midlife you may find yourself bound and restricted. The Western cultural model has firmly implanted a need for success in all of us, and our natural response has been to become rigid in the process.

But this attitude, which is stored in every cell of the body, does more harm than good. It can be the direct cause of degenerative illness, anxiety, and depression triggered by stress. A remarkable doctor told me once, "There is really only one illness, and it's stress, which manifests as everything from colds to heart disease. Stress also causes addictive habits, including drinking, smoking, and unhealthful diets that have a causative link to cancer and degenerative illness. Don't struggle with your habits. Just practice the Promise and see what happens to those imagined needs. The healing power flows inherently in you. We can successfully cope with and even need a certain amount of stress. We thrive on it, in fact. But not too much!"

Strength that is not receptive and cannot receive the feminine aspect is actually not strong at all. It is a vulnerable, brittle strength that breaks easily. When we become strong but can't receive, we shut down our engagement with life, effectively fencing ourselves in. Strength of this kind destroys itself, degenerating into illness and manifesting as a feeling of being at war with life, with yourself, and with everything else. And, of course, war is the ultimate degenerative illness.

The Promise will fix all this. The Promise is a soothing balm that starts with your self, moves through your family and community, and then to the whole world. You, your family, and finally everyOne are the benefactors of your Promise. Strength that is receiving makes ordinary strength stronger, more flexible, intelligent, and durable.

Sarah and Vishal:
The Promise of Procreation

Sarah and Vishal are a typical upwardly mobile couple who live a busy life, traveling frequently between New York and New Delhi. Vishal, who is Indian, has a successful Internet business in his homeland, while Sarah is an all-American girl who works as a designer and loves to keep fit by working out vigorously with popular styles of Yoga as it is taught in New York.

When Sarah turned thirty-six, she and Vishal decided to have a baby. They approached this, however, without interrupting their busy lives or changing their attitudes. Several years passed with no pregnancy. Finally, Sarah did conceive, only to miscarry early on. It had been a sad time for them, and, they admitted frankly, sex was not much fun.

At that point, a good friend of theirs called me in to help. I gave both Sarah and Vishal an appropriate practice: a variation on the Promise. Most important, I asked them to promise to practice nonobsessively but to do it at least once a day. I suggested that Sarah stop all overly assertive exercises, including her very aggressive Yoga routine, and find more time for leisure in a natural environment. And I asked Vishal to allow himself more time to enjoy his wife and to practice the Promise with her at home. With the special sexual practice of bypassing ejaculation until the period of Sarah's ovulation, Vishal maintained his intense desire, energy, and attention to her. Sarah loved that!

The immediate result was that their love, desire, and pleasure with each other increased dramatically. They were both more receptive to each other and more willing to make time for the simple pleasure of lovemaking. Sarah became more feminine in character and appearance, and so, more desirable to Vishal. In return, he became a little softer and less driven in his pursuit of business. Because of this, and his wife's increasing desirability, Vishal gave Sarah much more attention. Their lovemaking became more interesting to them, and they became more inventive with it. That may sound self-evident, but before doing the Promise, they had viewed sex almost as a job to be done—with the added pressure of trying to conceive.

And then, in the pleasure and health of their intimacy, that's precisely what happened. What joy they both felt! Sarah's belly grew beautifully, and when I saw them next, several months later, I was stunned by the radical change in how she looked in other ways. A thirty-eight-year-old tomboy had become a gracious woman; strong yet soft. It was amazing, because the mother force was also in her, and she was beautiful.

The Promise Is Promising

Underlying everything that you do in your life, you may feel a yearning for something deeper; something that will snap you out of your mundane reality and make you feel alive. And yet, paradoxically, this very search for something more implies that you don't *already* have what you're looking for. It implies that the ordinary body, breath, and sex are not enough, and so you have to keep looking.

Searching for enlightenment is a little like training to become an Olympic athlete. To make the Olympics, you need a high level of natural talent, a burning desire to succeed, and the stamina and persistence to train day in and day out. Many people apply the same intense effort to achieving a spiritual life. They believe that they have to spend hours a day in prayer, meditation, and other practices, often by sacrificing their family and even their professional career. They're afraid that if they miss a day or don't maintain a high level of practice, they'll backslide and lose all they've accomplished.

By contrast, the Promise is money in the bank; an absolutely secure investment that grows. You don't have to be a hero—and heroes often end up at zero! It's not obsessive, but it is cumulative. What you do today and tomorrow has implications for the future—for days, months, years, and even decades to come.

Indeed, this practice promises that you will be fulfilled, simply by having intimacy with your body and breath for several minutes a day. It doesn't matter what your particular passion or level of accomplishment is. Everyone can do this practice.

And it will fuel your other passions—languages, religions, culture, arts, and commerce—instead of draining your time and energy from them. All these will serve your intimate life, be an expression of it, and not take from it. If you like to surf or play music or cook or work as a life coach, it will make you a stronger surfer, a better musician, a more creative chef, a more effective coach.

The Promise will also intensify your personal relationships, including your intimate physical relationship with your special other. If your marriage, your primary partnership, is sagging under the weight of daily pressures, the Promise will breathe fresh air and energy back into it.

Jacquie: Intimacy, Not Enlightenment

Jacquie, who lives in Belgium, is a mother of two and a diplomat with the European Union. Her story is emblematic of many people who become so obsessed with seeking that they forget the basic things in life.

Until I learned the Promise, I found the lustful looks from my partner, including his sexual advances, to be a bit juvenile and, dare I say it, irritating. My perspective has changed so dramatically since then that it is hard to remember why I was so turned off, but let me try to revisit that mind-set.

For almost two decades, I've been a seeker, training my conscious mind with unwavering fervor. The discipline of all my enlightened practices, including meditation and self-help reading, has been both addictive and consuming. While I have enjoyed a clear understanding and awareness of my behavior, and have maintained an acute level of daily mindfulness, I realize how much I've been missing (including a wonderful sex life with my partner).

Now, I wouldn't go so far as to say that all my "self-discovery" work was turning me off sex per se, it just wasn't really turning me on—to anything, let alone my enthusiastic and ready-to-go partner. As I look back, I see that my lack of sexual interest was caused in large part by the fact that my mind was so preoccupied with watching my life that I was missing the most important part of life: experiencing it!

Conscious moving and breathing washes away the watcher in me like a wave washes away a crumbling, tired old sand castle. The practice of postures and breathing clears the decks and leaves me now ready, available, responsive, and welcoming. I feel I am stripping away my considerations and insights daily, and in this daily emptying, I am opening up. I am opening to a greater intimacy with myself, my wonderful partner, and our three lovely angels, who are five, four, and two years old. I am now seeing the truth of the message "When we stop looking, the natural state, which is love, seeps through." It doesn't get much simpler than that. Enjoy! It's why we're here.

By increasing your feeling of intimacy with yourself, the practice simultaneously opens you up to relating to others. You will have a renewed appreciation not merely for your individual passions but also for your sense of communion with others. Our heartbeat, breath, and sex are undeniably common to us all. It is the common ground. The intimacy is freely available, accessible by all, and gives fuel to everything else we want to achieve in life. It is a catalyst that brings forth all our possibilities; all our other intimate connections.

The Intervention:
Love Your Body as Yourself

Life is continually pulsing through your body, composing a magnificent symphony of various kinds of cells. Our bodies are infinitely complex, yet we rarely take time to stop and reflect on this wonder of nature. Unless something goes wrong, we assume that all the cells will continue doing their work. Right now, as you read these words, your body is performing the miracle of allowing you to breathe, function, and just exist.

Whether or not you are aware of it, you are involved in a constant relationship with life, one that is endlessly nurturing and sustaining. Consider how your body always operates with your best interests in mind—although not always in the best interests *of your mind*. The body always knows best. It works to heal you when you are ill and rewards you with energy and drive when you treat it kindly.

Once you accept that your body is inherently intuitive, you will see that life is a completely nurturing force, just as you trust that your bed will hold you when you sleep, and that the sun will rise in the morning. This is a simple but profound realization. Your intrinsic intelligence provides you with a life of unlimited intimacy, joy, and connection. Why? Because intimacy with your breath is intimacy with life. There is one life arising as yourself and with everyone and everything around you. You feel it. And the Source of it all. It is an utter pleasure.

Life offers infinite possibilities, and only your mind

imagines that your potential for realizing them is limited. Whenever you find yourself caught in cycles of negativity and doubt, which in most cases are simply responses to the pain of the world, you may imagine that love is beyond you. Sometimes it really does feel like life is an endless, unsupported struggle.

What you need is an intervention by someone who can throw you a rope and pull you out of the hole.

The great traditions deeply acknowledge that for a pattern to change, there must be an outside influence. In certain situations, we need something more extreme, such as a serious health scare, to shift our perspective and help us see what is really important. Or, an intervention may be necessary—such as when friends and family gather to help a loved one come to terms with a pattern of addictive behavior. The help we require may not be so drastic; it can be as subtle as gentle guidance from a friend, teacher, or mentor.

Think of the Promise as your own personal intervention. It is a call to realize that despite all the restrictions and impositions placed on you by society, culture, and religion, life stands alone. The practice that I will detail for you in the coming pages will allow you to let go of negative patterns and find a way of living that allows you to shed any restrictions that have been weighing you down and holding you back.

Your Source of Peace and Power

Whenever we approach anything new with a view to actualizing personal change and transformation, such as giving up smoking or starting a healthy diet, several factors determine whether or not we will be successful. It's normal to get carried away on the initial wave of enthusiasm, sharing our new convictions with everyone around us, only to see our resolve fall by the wayside a month later. While this initial motivation is vital, it is important to channel that excitement into our everyday lives in a realistic way.

Knowledge rests on the shelves of every bookcase, and is encoded in millions of websites and computers. Yet the secret lies not in knowledge but in the wisdom of your own life, which has already been given to you. The secrets of the universe are already in you *as you*. You are formed from the very substance and the mystery processes of the universe. We are all made of stars!

Different cultures and spiritual traditions express this truth in different terms. Some speak of Buddha nature, meaning that your True Self is embedded under layers of conditioned identity, waiting to be set free. Others refer to the presence of God in each of us. Or they say that the vessel of the Light originally shattered into billions of shards, and every human being is illuminated by one of these fragments. None of these images or conceptions explains fully what I mean.

Let me put it this way: the extreme intelligence and

beauty of life are functioning in you *as you already are*. The intelligence of male-female polarity, which can create new life, down to even the way your skin functions, is an unfathomable intelligence that science cannot understand. You *are* Nurturing Source Reality. No attempt to know consciousness will achieve it. You already *are* that consciousness, so *no* looking is required—just participating in what is already given.

What Is Male-Female Polarity, Anyway?

Let me take a moment here to explain what I mean by male-female polarity, and why it's essential to the underlying principles of the Promise. I discuss this in more depth later, as part of a larger concept that we call the union of opposites, but you need to understand the basic premise here.

The union of opposites is the intrinsic method of our universe by which all things appear, sustain, and regenerate. In the close observations of science, we see atoms and molecules and cells functioning as the poles of negative and positive energy, utterly attracted and attached to one another in precise form. In our most expansive view, we see the grand orchestration of suns and planets moving in the same attraction of opposite poles holding one another in the mystery patterns of known and unknown stars. An intelligence, function, and beauty is operating in the world we know that is beyond comprehension. That same intelligence is also present in our human life in each beautiful person, in heartbeat, in breath, and in sex. This attraction of opposites, the male-female equation of life, is how we all got here. It continues to move as the absolute power of life that sustains us all, and renews and improves the species. This is the nurturing flow of the universe and is the secret to longevity.

The male and female qualities are present as the essential nature of all opposites, such as left and right, above and below, dark and light, inhalation and exhalation. It is as simple as that. By participating in the union of all ordinary opposite poles, the male-female qualities of "strength that is receptive" are permitted to flourish in social life. And most astonishingly, the source of opposites—this nurturing force and function of our universe— is perceived. We know the eternal power that is presently operating as our human form. Sex, the utter union of male and female, instantly created your mother and father and brought you into form. Sex is not an obstruction to knowing our source but the very means of knowing it. The Promise shows us how to participate in the opposites in every way. It shows us how to intelligently enjoin the power of life and sex in a most positive and wonder-full way. It is a priceless gift that reveals your peace, power, and purpose.

Yet that same power also exists in your very breath, and in the combination of breath and movement that is at the heart of the Promise Practice. What you truly need is not secret knowledge but a realistic practice that will allow you to navigate through the noise and chaos in your life, and direct you to the source of peace and power that is in you. The practice is not intended as a quick bite of daily escapism or a shortcut to transcendence. Not a trick, something to do in your room each day to feel a little better. Instead it is participation in the whole of life. It is designed as a grounded distillation of all that is: something that occurs naturally when you create an opening that allows the peace and happiness already within you to arise. Contradictory as it may seem, the practice is more a path of relaxation than of action, relaxing into what life is. It is a catalyst that releases all of your potential. Think of a piece of cork held down by a large rock at the bottom of a lake. When you remove the rock, the cork will bob to the surface of its own accord. Similarly, the Promise removes obstructions to your experience of happiness and peace, allowing these qualities to fill your entire being. What manifests when you undertake the practice may be subtle or dramatic, but is entirely personal. It is your gift to yourself.

Bob's Story: Singing to the Toaster

When I first met Bob Dolman (who wrote the foreword), he was having difficulty coming to terms with his busy, driven life. He was doing what he had to get done, but he was feeling disconnected from the source of his real power. The practice described in this book has helped Bob gain intimacy with the core of his being while he continues to go about the daily business of his work and his relationships.

When I wake up in the morning, some ambitious part of me is waiting by the bed with a list of things to do. If I do them all, evidently, I'll become someone amazing. This has been going on for decades. Usually I do everything on the list, but lately I've been beginning the day by breathing and moving, easily and enjoyably, without any agenda at all. I am more present in my body, with a physical confidence that encourages openness and fearless dissolving. That is, the armor that I have built up over a lifetime is chipping off, and I'm able to go to smithereens—blissfully—and know that I won't disintegrate altogether.

There's even wholeness on the other side of wild abandon, and to trust that after doubting it for so long is a big and beautiful step. Don't ask me how it works, but the lemon tree looks incredible, and the woman I live with is singing to the toaster. I spend the rest of the day doing less and accomplishing more. And the amazing person I'm supposed to become, I found out a minute ago, has been sitting here on the sunporch strumming a ukulele.

The Promise Practice allows you to relax and fully enjoy your life, while appreciating all that surrounds you. This is intimacy in the most profound sense. And what exactly do we mean by "intimacy"?

In the context of the Promise, intimacy refers to a heightened sense of perception and intelligence, both sensory and emotional, which moves you toward ease and truth, and can be both sexual and nonsexual. This intimacy involves enjoying the sound of auburn leaves crunching under your feet, the quiet patch of coolness beneath tree branches, and the warmth of your lover's body wrapped around you in a jigsaw puzzle of skin.

A woman who attended one of my workshops reported a mystifying experience. After years of doing so-called spiritual practices, including meditations, chanting, and various physical exercises, she started doing the Promise. "Suddenly," she said, "one morning after doing the Promise, I noticed the lamp shade on my night table. Now, that lamp shade had been on the lamp next to my bed for so many years, but I hadn't really noticed it before. And it was beautiful. I saw every inch and aspect of its design, the way the light filtered through it and changed colors, the way it warmed the entire room with its simple glow."

In moments like these, we love being alive. Finding intimacy starts inside, the mind becomes clear, and the barriers between you and the beauty all around you dissolve. Caught up in the stress of everyday life, work, family, and relationships, we often find it hard to stop, relax, and appreciate the lemon tree. Living in a society fueled by consumerism, constant stimulation, instant gratification, or too many cups of coffee, our natural state has effectively been hijacked. We need the practical tools to reclaim it on a daily basis.

Consider Cynthia's experience of how conscious breath and movement helped her overcome her anxiety:

When I stop, or even slow down, I notice how frantic my mind and energy have become. I'm not even really breathing. I have so many things "to do," it feels like I'm not really in my body. I don't even taste my food. I'm madly efficient and then madly lost. I used to be like that a lot. I just thought it was normal, even though I was "holding it together." I looked happy, with a successful life, but often I'd feel anxious, lonely, and depressed inside. Then I started to breathe. When I began practicing the Promise, I saw how different things could be. In my body, when I started breathing, I began finding a place where I knew everything was okay—and more than that. I not only felt my body but also a source of peace and strength emanating from within it.

With the help of these practices, you will start to recognize intimacy in its infinitely beautiful form as your daily life. You will see that you have everything you need at this very moment, regardless of your personal circumstances, your job, how much money you earn or don't earn, how many children you have or don't have, or your past experiences.

We all have the ability to connect to our breath and relax into our natural state.

CHAPTER 3

Stop Looking, Start Living

Seeking anything implies that you don't have it. The very action denies your intrinsic reality. The world has been seduced by the idea of enlightenment. Your search negates the truth that is you, as you already are, the present embodiment of life's wonder—a living, breathing expression of reality itself.

OUR FIRST WORLD PROBLEMS HAVE LED US TO A PLACE where we seem to need some ancient wisdom to sort them out. Having realized the myth of the materialistic dream, it has become an appealing option for many people to investigate other ways of looking at the world. In the process, so-called enlightenment has been presented as a convincing antidote to the dissatisfaction and impermanence of our materially driven lives. Because of this, the self-help industry is now worth billions of dollars. The popular fascination with Zen, yoga, meditation, and a myriad of related spiritual practices indicates a genuine desire for greater self-awareness and personal development. But the mass marketing of inner peace is not always benign. Often in this search to find a solution to the ills of modern life, we get caught in a compulsive cycle, not dissimilar to the very thing from which we were trying to break free!

The truth is that most of us aren't actually looking to transcend life but to enjoy the life we do have more fully. Our Western lifestyles are so oriented toward work, achievement, and material success that taking time is still viewed as a luxury. Our lunchtime conversations often revert to shared stories about life's struggles. What we all seem to be seeking is to improve our lives and to gain a greater sense of peace. The question remains, though, *how* do we get it?

In many cases, the solutions we come up with require money, which often has negative connotations in the context of a spiritual search. When you come to see money as a natural flow and exchange of energy, however, you can view it as an integral part of Nurturing Source Reality. When you develop a healthy relationship with money, in order to take care of yourself and the people you love, a natural economy arises, and money ceases to be an object of power, greed, and fear. It is simply the flow of Nurturing Source. The way you spend it, and the things you choose to spend it on, will reflect the expression of your values, and if you do this, you have no need to fear money. The line from Scripture that is often misquoted as "Money is the root of all evil" actually says, "The love of money is the root of all kinds of evil" (1 Timothy 6:10). Money itself is not the issue, but the obsessive fixation with money is.

The uneasy relationship with money is only part of the issue, though. What is causing people even greater suffering is the merchandising of inner peace. The great wisdom teachings have been marketed as impossible ideals for those of us living "normal" lives. The concept of enlightenment, for example, has been offered as a state of stark contrast to the lives we are actually living. We hear that a world of spiritual joy awaits us, but meanwhile, we are bound to the routines of working, studying, having relationships, raising children, and washing the dishes.

No matter how hard you try to be the enlightened observer, to stand outside the stream of daily life and view it objectively, the demands of domesticity require engaging with this material world. The dishes do not wash themselves. Yet popular spiritual teachers have presented everyday aspects of life—the normal activities of sex, family, work, and relationships—as merely the content of your awareness training or, worse, an obstruction to it. This is a mistake. These seemingly mundane activities are themselves the all-powerful means to achieving greater consciousness. This may humorously remind you of the words of the renowned African-American preacher known as Reverend Ike, who used to rail against religions that urged followers to wait for what he called "pie in the sky by-and-by when you die." Ike thought that you should have your abundance right now, right here on earth! And in his own way, he was right.

In the process of trying to attain some heightened sense of being, the spiritual equivalent of pie in the sky, you can end up feeling hungrier than ever, especially when you fail to achieve or sustain your chosen state of stillness. Feeling inadequate, instead of enlightened, is an inevitable result of this dichotomy. Paradoxically, then, the very search for the idea of enlightenment leads you further away from it. Get it? By implying that enlightenment is missing you, you come to believe that you are lacking something you need to be truly happy and at peace.

It's like trying to find your keys. You know they were definitely around; you had them just ten minutes ago. But they're not on the table, on the couch, or in the car. Where are they?! You rummage, fumble, and curse until you finally realize the obvious. They were in your pocket all along! Or have you ever wasted time looking for your glasses only to find them on top of your head? You feel bemused, relieved, and happy. Not looking anymore! You just got so absorbed in the search that you stopped seeing straight.

Amy's Story:
Slowing Down and Listening

Amy Hansen is a thirty-nine-year-old physician who had just spent a year in Alaska "getting in touch with" herself when we met. By her own account, she was pouring so much time and energy into an unending search for enlightenment that she was having difficulty relating to her family—and to other people, including potential romantic partners—on a human level.

I'd never had luck with intimacy in partnership, and I was using spiritual practices to escape from engaging in life. I had been abused sexually as a child, and, not surprisingly, didn't have very nurturing parents. As a result, I felt abandoned. And because I didn't love myself, I did things to escape from myself.

Perhaps because I was really scared of what was inside me, I was constantly trying to grasp for outside things to make myself feel better. In my search for enlightenment, I always thought that I needed to keep doing more and more to "get somewhere." I read every book, went to every retreat. I wanted to believe that I was already perfect—that I was God; that everyone was God. But I was still highly critical of myself. That's when I started doing the Promise.

The first thing that happened was that I started really checking in with myself. I noticed my breathing more, and the breath became the focus of the practice. Instead of trying to control life, I softened to what life was offering me. I opened up to the world, inviting creativity in the form of dance, song, and all relationships. For the first time in my life, I accepted and loved vulnerability. I finally had no desire to sit like a monk in a cave. Instead I wanted to engage in relationship with others. I no longer felt guarded, afraid that interactions would drain me.

I sank into my feminine nature, and that allowed the nurturing current to run through me, so that it could be shared with others in conversation, at work, and finally in a relationship. I had started doing the Promise three months prior to meeting my partner. One month after we started seeing each other, I got pregnant! As I carry the baby inside of me, now I am experiencing an intimacy that I could not have imagined.

I will admit that with the new relationship and the pregnancy, I have been pushed to my limit, and at times I start to go back into old patterns. And yet this has shown me the importance of doing my breathing. When I get scared about the future, I have this intimacy with myself, and I know how to care for myself. And the simple practice, focused on inhaling and exhaling, following wisdom that naturally exists by having a body, has allowed me to surrender. I still have a tendency to try to control things when fear sneaks in, but the practice, the relationship with myself, softens me. I can be still amidst the storm. Pregnancy has been a great teacher. It is my practice at this time—and it is not separate from the Promise. I have discussed with my partner that the Promise is a commitment to ourselves and to each other to stay engaged and maintain the intimacy. We want to show up for each other and for our child. It helps to quiet the mind, and helps me listen to life, to what the universe is offering.

The Source and Seen Are One!

Deeply embedded in the religious philosophies of the ancient world was the idea of a Source Reality that manifests as the universe in all its detail. Later cultures used the words *God, Yahweh, Allah,* or *Lord,* among others, to express this Source concept. World religions were formed around this idea, each expressing in its unique way that the Creator and creation are one.

As time passed, however, people lost connection with this initial truth. New doctrines persuaded followers to *search* for the Source, as if it were not present in the very substance of everything.

The logical outcome of this was to deny or exploit ordinary reality in an attempt to get to the almighty Source.

This has been going on for millennia: the belief that God is "up there" in heaven, while we struggle "down here" on Earth. All manner and means of seeking arose, as if Truth or God or Source were somehow absent. Today searching for truth has become an uninspected habit, a cosmic game of hide-and-seek that we are all supposed to play.

Instead let's look back at the original belief that Source and seen really are the same. There is no difference between spirit and matter. It's like trying to separate day and night—without one, the other cannot exist. This idea may encourage you to reevaluate the whole notion of *seeking* truth. When you stop seeking, you create an opportunity to become intimate with that truth. Intimate with the Divine. Intimate with the ordinary conditions of life. Intimate with your self. They are all one and the same, as readily available as your breath.

The habit of discontent, of obsessively looking and waiting for something outside yourself, can be discarded altogether. When you do this, you will be free to start living in truth; in what is. For me, that means the reality that is always upon us in every breath, every heartbeat, and every relationship.

And that is the end of the story. You are already in Source Reality, and the extreme intelligence of all life is streaming forth continuously. "Stop looking, start living!" The spiritual life is one of participation only in what is— not an endless search. It is intimacy, here and now, with body and breath. From this starting point, this intimacy with your self, every other intimate action is easily within your grasp. You no longer dissociate from your circumstances. You choose intimacy with reality and all its detail. You taste life!

The moment you reestablish a connection to your Source, all outside influences become expressions of happiness and well-being instead of futile attempts to achieve it. From here, you are open and free enough to deal with whatever presents itself to you, supported by the knowledge that this intimate connection with your source of strength and truth is all that is required to feel safe and at peace.

The Promise is a simple practice of breathing and movement that will help you establish a life of intimacy with yourself and others.

Source Reality

The essence of this most profound universal truth is contained within the following two concise questions. Be still for a moment, let go of all previous assumptions and associations as much as you can, and consider them with an open mind.

1. Is the life that is your body, heartbeat, and breath an extreme intelligence, function, and beauty that is beyond scientific understanding? Yes or no?
2. If there is such a thing as an unseen source of this intelligence, can it ever be absent from its visibility and intelligence that is you? Yes or no?

I am not asking these as spiritual questions. They are not an attempt at existential poetry. This is math; the pure logic of existence. Use the visual image of an iceberg to understand this. Although you see only the tip of the iceberg, you intuitively know that there is far more under the water's surface. The Source of life is no different. What you see and experience *as you* in your life on earth is just the tip of the iceberg. Yet you are intimately connected to all of it.

If you answered yes to the first question, you agree that you are indeed an infinite, intelligent, and beautiful expression of life. And if you answered no to the second, then you acknowledged that it is impossible for you to be separated from that Source Reality, or for it ever to be absent. In which case, you can now relax. You *are* the wonder of life.

The true magnificence of life does not await you. It is not pie in the sky by-and-by; it actually *is* you. When you came out of your mother's womb, your family was brought to its knees, staggered by the mystery. It blew their minds to meet you. From where did you come? How could this be? They marveled as they looked into your eyes that revealed infinity.

It is still true, however many years into life you are. You are the utter wonder of reality itself, and here you are. We should all be brought to our knees to see each other in the wonder that is our life!

The Ordinary Is Extraordinary

We all need to connect. But intimacy with another is not possible until you experience intimacy with your own life. The starting point of intimacy is with your own body and breath. As you begin to engage the body in unison with the breath, you develop an inner sensitivity and receptivity that, in turn, allow you to receive another intimately. The practice of physical movement with synchronized breath allows you the necessary internal sensitivity to develop intimate relationships. You then begin to feel your own connectedness with everything around you, including the deep and absolute intimacy provided by life that forms the basis of everything.

In order for this realization to flower, all you need to do is initiate your practice of moving and breathing for seven minutes a day to support the energetic flow of life through your system. As you do, the veil that causes a feeling of separateness and isolation will be lifted, revealing the naked wonder of your own natural state. What results is a beautiful adventure with life.

Amanda Harberg, Concert Pianist

Amanda was having health issues that were interfering with her career as a concert pianist. She had been struggling to compose and perform using all the technical complexities that she had derived from her academic musical education at the prestigious Juilliard School. The stress of performing at the edge of her technical capability was compounding the pain in her back and arms, making it even more difficult to create freely and easily, whether while playing or composing new music. Her spirits had been low, her marriage strained, and she had serious doubts about her career.

At the time I started working with Amanda, she had not begun dabbling in spiritual techniques or meditation methods, so it was easy to teach her a physical practice that might otherwise have conflicted with her preconceptions. By doing a simple moving and breathing practice each day, she was able to discover her own breath and life, and once she relaxed into her life, her physical and emotional pain eased and eventually dissipated.

Further, as an extension of her daily practice of the Promise, I asked her to go to the piano each day and play purely for her own pleasure, without pushing technical boundaries. The results were astonishing for herself and everybody else. As her breath and body moved just like life, so did her music. Amanda began to experience a new level of success as a performer and a renewed career as a composer. New, high-quality work flowed from her spontaneously. Her compositions became an expression of who she is and how she feels, unrestricted by technique or preconceived musical styles. Her music touched a new depth, and new life came through her hands.

As a bonus, Amanda began to love her life, especially the intimacy with her husband. Nor was that something separate, like taking a course or working with a marriage or sex counselor. It arose spontaneously, along with her new freedom of composing and performing.

At a dinner party some months later, I had the pleasure of hearing Amanda perform her new piano compositions. They were beautiful, full of feeling and yet peaceful. She told all of us that she had found a new depth of simplicity in composing. Although she didn't explain the connection to those present at the party, the significance of her new pieces wasn't lost on me. They are titled "Breathing Songs."

The Promise is a catalyst to activate your creative or career aspirations. By relaxing and being intimate with your own body and breath, you naturally become more intimate with your own creative activity—be it art, music, or raising your children.

I suggest that you too find time each day to enjoy your particular creative pastime, whether that takes the form of painting, gardening, swimming, cooking, walking, or any of the myriad activities that you can enjoy without imposing any particular criteria to measure your success or failure.

Do it for its own sake because you love it.

CHAPTER 4

On Earth as It Is in Heaven

You do not need to step back from your experience and curb your natural desires in order to find and know God. Connecting to your spiritual ideals through your own body and breath is a positive process that will assure you of your own power and strength, and free you from the struggle to attain another level of being than that which is your natural condition.

No DOUBT AT SOME POINT YOU HAVE ASKED YOURSELF, Is there a God? And if not, then what? We've been grappling with the mystery of why we're here and what we're supposed to be doing since the beginning of human history.

However you answer these questions is entirely personal. You may be a member of a particular religion, and so you base your life on its teachings to some degree. Or you may feel cynical about all notions of faith. Perhaps the mention of God or anything spiritual leaves you fearful of what that means and represents.

Regardless of your beliefs, the desire for connection is

present within all of us. We all seek ways to break down the barriers between ourselves and others. Our means and motivations are not always spiritual. An after-work ritual of gathering at the bar to loosen the body and tongue with drinks is a modern version of the ancient campfire and stargazing. Our sense of identity and worth, and the values we come to hold, all grow out of our relationships. The importance of our interdependence cannot be overstated. We crave the closeness of other human beings.

Our ancestors perceived the universe as a vast, integrated force that encompassed everything that they could see, touch, and feel, as well as all that exists within the intangible, or subtle, realms. Underlying all this, they taught, is the absolute Source of life—the sustaining, nurturing, and regenerating force.

But they also recognized that the toil and survival needs of the everyday world made it difficult for people to acknowledge themselves as manifestations of this same Spirit or Source. The concept of interdependence could be lost. And so the ancient masters developed *practices* to combat the illusion that people were separate from the earth, separate from those around them, and separate from their Source. These everyday practices were shared freely so that this truth could blossom inside of everyone. They formed the foundation from which all other religious and spiritual life arose. The intention of these practices was simple but magnificent: to establish an unending intimacy with life and form within everyday, ordinary existence.

This same intention, or Promise, is being offered to you now. I am writing this book in order to pass the ancient practices along to you so that you can implement them in your life in a simple and joyful way, and by doing so, tap into the intimacy of your own body and breath, and improve your intimacy and interconnectedness with others.

Reverend Reho's Story

The Reverend Dr. James H. Reho ministered to a congregation at Trinity Episcopal Cathedral in Miami, Florida, where he developed an experimental Eucharistic service, led multiple retreats, and gave forums on spiritual practice in a pluralistic world. Sometime after he began doing the Promise, Reverend Reho was appointed chaplain and director of pastoral care, deployment, and formation at the General Theological Seminary in New York. The minister's experience shows that, irrespective of your religious and spiritual convictions, the practices you will draw from the Promise can coexist seamlessly with your beliefs:

The day after having "promised" to practice this short sequence, I had a beautiful experience. About twenty minutes after completing this simple routine, I was sitting on my couch, reading and having a snack, and I felt my heart open in an exhilarating, profound way. I experienced myself and everything around me flooded with love and joy. I had a great desire to share this love with everyone around me, and also a profound understanding that the entire universe was already, beautifully, enveloped in it. I saw the unity of all love—spiritual, emotional, and sexual—and felt divinely opened to love even more deeply in each of these aspects of life. It was a moment of my eyes and heart being opened, a deep communion with God/the Divine.

As an Episcopal priest, I later reflected on how my own tradition teaches that God is love, and how Jesus taught that the kingdom of God is here, spread out before us, and our "work" is to open our minds and hearts to that love. This practice, accessible to everyone, helps in that work. My hope is that more and more people, of every faith tradition, will make the promise to practice these teachings, and as a result will come to experience more and more that our world and everyone in it is brimming with immanent, divine love.

Reverend Reho is right: there is heaven on earth!

My Islamic and Jewish Friends

For the past five years, I've been participating in a nonprofit organization that trains and nurtures aspiring teachers from conflict zones around the world, regardless of their ability to pay. The training gives them the tools and techniques necessary to teach others the Promise Practice. Teachers interpret these teachings in a way that makes sense in their home country, and don't contradict or supplant indigenous religious and cultural customs and beliefs.

The results have been extraordinary, especially in the Middle East, where they have brought together Islamic and Jewish women by teaching simple yet powerful physical practices. Islam is one of the few institutional religions that engage in "whole body prayer" on an everyday basis. Indeed, orthodox Muslims pray five times daily, and their prayers are connected to a series of precise physical movements. Several Muslim women who have learned the Promise Practice report that it has greatly enhanced their engagement in and appreciation of the conventional Muslim prayers they already perform every day. The classes also often involve Muslim and Jewish women learning the practice together.

Here is one account from a Muslim woman who had been taking classes in East Jerusalem. (Because of political conditions there, her identity has been withheld.)

I teach Koranic studies to women in the East Jerusalem community. Over the last few years, I have been attending breath and movement classes with both Jewish and Muslim women in our neighborhood. In our class, we end every lesson in a heart circle where we all hold hands and connect hearts, connect to the love, and then send it out to where it is needed—to the suffering and trauma in East and West Jerusalem, Israel, and Palestine. These classes have helped me feel more connected to an infinite source of love, even though we are surrounded by pain. I pray deeper. I love deeper, and I want to teach the women in my class how to adapt these principles to their daily prayers so they can connect to God directly from their hearts. I know it will keep us strong and together. The Promise Practice combined with our five-times-daily prayer cycle has helped me personally feel the depth of our faith of love. It has become my joy to pray, rather than just a social duty.

Her prayer practice changed from being an exoteric duty to an esoteric or personal connection to life and truth. This story shows so clearly how the connections that are formed through the union of body and breath with each other offer us the experience of divinity. This isn't done through some contrived performance, or through a denial of the Given Reality. Instead a powerful connection to breath, body, and *others* is fundamental to these sacred, transformative experiences. It belongs in all the world faiths as the practical means to realize their beautiful ideals. Nurturing Source Reality is acknowledged as being alive and present in each person.

This is the underlying principle within this book, and I want to make sure that it is established at this early point. What you may have been seeking in the various forms of spiritual practice that now abound is available to you right now, and you do not have to deny yourself the full experience of life in order to get it. You do not need to forgo intimacy and involvement with other people. You do not need to repress or mask the full wonder of yourself in any way at all! What I will show you in the following chapters is that all the wonderful spiritual ideals that you may have read about or thought about will actually become a living reality for you through the Promise Practice.

But the key word here is *practice.*

Bringing the ideas and philosophies of faith into material form is not an impossible dream. As we saw with our Islamic and Jewish friends, we can make a start in the midst of arduous social conditions. It is my hope for humanity that we can celebrate our common life, our breath, our families, and also celebrate our unique differences as individuals and cultures.

From Lisa Shalom, a Young Jewish Activist and Environmentalist

When I turned twenty, I left home to join a conservation ship, the Ocean Warrior, *and "save the world." I felt that indulging in anything other than radical direct action would be inappropriate on a planet in the midst of ecocide. My outward mission eventually turned to inward seeking, as I eventually reached a point of exhaustion at trying to change everything that didn't fit my understanding of justice. I began to realize that the beast I had real access to taming lay under my very own skin. At about age twenty-three, I began to practice the Promise and Judaism, with sincerity, commitment, and a newfound understanding that inward focus and practice were not only more satisfying for the soul but also simply more effective at influencing the world around me positively.*

Rather than surfacing as a source of conflict, my Promise Practice has greatly informed my Judaism and vice versa. Among others points of commonality is Shabbat—Saturday, the Jewish day of rest, which is very much about absorbing the Shekinah, or the presence of the feminine attributes of God. Every Friday, along with Jewish women around the world, I light two candles, sing, bless wine, break bread with friends and family, and we make time to be together and discuss our valuable "lessons of the week." It's a process of settling into what is, taking time to

be with it, bringing awareness to the subtleties of life, and slow-
ing down to connect to ourselves, each other, and God, just as
the Promise Practice helps me to do. Both my Promise Practice
and my Judaism call for a deep acknowledgment and acceptance
of the now, without resistance.

In Hebrew, the word for breath and the word for soul are
written using the same letters: neshima (נשימה) *and* neshama
(נשמה). *The breath is an offering of life from an intangible
force, which cannot be seen or defined. It is a gift that comes
freely on its own with birth. In a very real way, it's our link to the
source of creation, to the Divine, just as the soul is considered in
Judaism to be a spark, or a piece of this source, of God.*

So when I intentionally invite my breath to fill me with a vital
life force, as done in the Promise Practice, I am tuning into that
which exists beyond my perception, and of which I am innately
a part. When I allow the breath to guide my movement, I give
myself to this divine wisdom, which creates my existence inside
of each passing moment. Within the experience of the Promise,
it becomes clear that the breath of life wants to give itself, the
earth wants to cradle, the sky wants to support. This process
of allowing is a big one for me in my Promise Practice, as within
my Judaism.

I was born with the last name Shalom, meaning "peace" in
Hebrew, which is also used as a popular form of greeting in the
Jewish world. The word shalom and the Promise, when practiced, are both embodiments of union. Peace and the Promise
both require coexistence of opposites to bloom. Through the
union of opposites, I know my Source. In order to rise, I need to
root. In order to have peace, I need only participate in the union
of opposites.

A Promise That Delivers

Since humankind developed the written word and was able to create abstract meaning, promises were given of the sublime experiences that were possible in human life. These were simply descriptions of intimate realization that had occurred naturally throughout the ancient world as humanity experienced its direct intimacy with Reality through every kind of connection to the natural state. With the development of the written word, such experience became defined in text, which became doctrine, and the worldwide hierarchy, or priesthood, was presumed to have and give access to the sublimity described in its texts. However, all that remained were abstract idealisms and man's desire for these possibilities, without the practical means by which union with the absolute was felt in the first place. Doctrine as abstraction and institution had stripped intimacy with all ordinary conditions from its teachings and was presenting beautiful ideals, creating desire in humanity without giving the actual means.

This is why incorporating the Promise into your life will deliver the actual hopes and messages that are the basis of religious institutions in the ancient and contemporary worlds. This is the promise that delivers those promises. It also delivers on all the promises given to us in the modern commercial world—including every kind of potion and pill that clever marketing has manipulated us to believe will make us healthy, sexy, beautiful, and blissful. All the while, we are ignoring the plain wonder, extreme intelligence, and function of our natural state. In the Promise, we let the wonder and utter connection to life be sufficient. We let breath be sufficient. We let this sitting here be sufficient. We let the Reality be sufficient. We enjoy the intrinsic, inborn powers of life moving in us. Life itself moves us into every kind of wonderful relatedness, including deep, abiding sexual intimacy freely chosen in the way that is right for us as individuals.

So let's not throw out the baby with the bathwater. The Promise is the anciently given means that enables us to realize the wonderful ideals expressed in the languages of faith. This tiny addition gives us the clarity that all faiths are simply different cultural expressions of the same human wonder. The different faiths are brought together, and even the atheist and the theist embrace in the tangible depth of life and breath. We bloom where we have been planted in our own garden. This is my Promise to you.

CHAPTER 5

Intimacy with Life in All Forms

Ordinary life is not just about the self. If it were, we should not have survived long as a species. The interrelationship among all things and all beings is fundamental to this journey we are on, and should be celebrated.

For most people, life does not look like a neat and ordered event. Quite the opposite, in fact. It appears as a complex patchwork of relationships, commitments, and activities. Even when the life we live has a certain structure to it, the nature of it is often chaotic. The flow of life moves through different contexts of work, family, friends, partners, and children, and issues and dramas arise inevitably. Society asks us to be highly adept at dealing with constantly changing circumstances. We all play many different roles during the space of a single day and wear various social masks.

Yet it is in this complexity that the wonder of our life resides if we choose to engage with it. The most ordered existence still contains elements of surprise, urging us to remain open, adaptable, and receptive.

Our modern way of life asks a lot of us, though, so we often question how we will keep ourselves in some sort of balance. Everyday life looks and feels so vastly different from what is presented as ideal through popular media: the lives of entertainers, celebrities, politicians, athletes, corporate titans, and millionaires of all stripes. These impossibly high, manufactured standards contribute to our belief that our own lives are somehow less than ideal and that happiness must lie somewhere else. Often our thoughts center on how life would be if circumstances were better, and we put off making changes because we don't feel that they are possible.

Yet our refusal to embrace the nurturing power of our given reality is at the heart—the real source—of what causes all our suffering. The inability to accept and embrace what is given to us as something entirely sacred, even in the most minor way, breeds an attitude of denial and ignorance that is harmful to us and those around us. It might be worth considering how you feel about your own life, as it is given. Are you satisfied with it and intimately connected to it? Or do you still privately subscribe to the mythical idea that life is "out there" or "in here," waiting for you to arrive?

If you can, recall the last time that you unashamedly enjoyed a moment of honest gratitude for yourself and the wonder of being alive. Not just in a theoretical or abstract way, but including your physical body, your unique personality, and all your relationships. Most of us are so overly concerned with the stresses of what is happening each day of the coming week, month, and even year that we're unable to indulge in the luxury of simple appreciation for what is already available to us. Life seems like a continual balancing act between work, family, and relationships. But how much of this time do we really value and enjoy?

Shelley's Story: Eat, Pray, Run Away

Dr. Shelley Cowden has a PhD in philosophy. She wandered into a workshop of mine while traveling in Bali, and learned to move and breathe freely. This is her account:

After losing love and a relationship that I had hoped would be long term, I was washed up financially and emotionally. The sense of dread about my future was totally consuming. Not one single thing in my life gave me joy. I felt that the only possible way my pain and disconnection from life would be healed was if I could just get to my real self, and to God. However, as I felt at the time, both of these things were far removed from my disastrous life. I believed that I needed to go to an exotic and "spiritual" location that would allow me to reconnect with my True Self. I ran far away to India and Asia and obsessively sat in all the holy places I could find. I lit incense at every temple and kneeled before every Buddha. But something still didn't feel right.

Added to this was the bizarre coincidence that my holiday

book was a copy of Eat, Pray, Love, *given to me by a coworker.*
Inspired by the story, I pressed on in my search, feeling abso-
lutely confident that it would indeed work for me too! I felt it
was a sign that I had found the perfect "runaway recipe"! I
chanted on the banks of the Ganges, climbed sacred mountains,
and worshipped every god and goddess statue I could find. Surely
this was a path to some higher reality where my hurt would
disappear and I would magically transcend the oh-so-human
conditions of pain, suffering, and loss that still plagued me. You
can imagine my disappointment to find that I was wrong. It
seemed like a bad dream. I just could not find what I was looking
for. Lit more incense. More hoping. More moping. More medita-
tion. More looking.

But then my money ran out, and my travels came to a
sad end. I had to return to my life at home in Australia and
pretend to everyone that I was okay. My mind was so dark it
scared me. So in total desperation, I thought I would give the
Eat, Pray, Love formula one last try by running to Bali for a
spiritual festival. Wrong again. While standing stiffly among
scantily clad gymnasts, trying to readjust my stance to mimic
their stoic commitment to the perfect posture, I couldn't help
but feel worse. I was fighting back tears of despair as I made
my way to my last workshop for the day. Within this space, I
was introduced to a practice that changed everything. Within
a few minutes, this one teacher made me feel what I had been
seeking for months.

It seemed too easy, but the simple connection of my breath
with my body movement, something he called Your Seven-
Minute Wonder, released me from the isolation, suffering, and
unhappiness that had become my reality. I felt okay to cry. My

chest stopped hurting. I stopped thinking about everything that was wrong and realized that my life as it was, despite the pain and trauma, was all exactly as it needed to be. Maybe my life didn't look the way I had imagined it would when I started out, but it was still all right. Even after losing the person I thought would be my life partner, I could feel whole. In the simple act of acknowledging my own self as the main spiritual event, everything started to shine again. The practice led me through my own physical experience of reality, and I realized that once my body and breath connected, everything else began to connect again as well. It was something I could take home, and I didn't need to go anywhere to find it. I could stop running. Since then, it has been a continual part of my life, and I have no fear of this promise being broken.

The Pull of Familial Bonds

The first experience we have of relationship is through the nurturing power of family, and this often forms the bedrock for our growth and expansion in life. Through the union of mother and father—the male-female polarities—we are given life. All family connections spring from this coupling, and life itself is dependent entirely on the continued merger of male and female energies.

At the same time, the roles of mothers and fathers, aunts and uncles, grandparents, siblings, and cousins can also be thoroughly confusing, especially in the modern world, where separations, stepfamilies, and broken homes are common. One way we tend to respond is by inhibiting expressions of love and affection among family members.

Emily's Story: A Way of Healing

I've always had a good relationship with my father, but, of course, with normal events in life, there can be some distancing. I knew I wanted to change this, but I wasn't sure what to do about it. I had taken up the Promise as a way of healing for myself after a troubled time, and I found that through it, I was able to reconnect with some of the pain from my childhood.

In particular, I started working through stored grief from the death of my mother at an early age. I finally stopped fighting with the sadness and allowed myself to feel it as inhale and exhale, letting it move through me rather than holding on and causing restrictions in myself. When I acknowledged the reality of the sad feelings within myself, it also enabled me to see the reality of how my father had felt and why he reacted in certain ways. It dawned on me that most of the sadness and pain we feel with loss are tied up in fighting against those emotions instead of letting ourselves feel.

This process was so beneficial that I encouraged my dad to start as well, and now he too does the Seven-Minute Wonder every morning. We have practiced together at times and often share our experiences of the Promise very openly. As a result, our conversation is often on the same wavelength, because we are both balancing the male and female polarities within ourselves. A lot of the misunderstandings we used to have are now less frequent or totally resolved. The little niggling issues that

used to be a problem seem so much less important than honest
communication and love, and there is so much more of that
now. I think the Promise has played a big part in strengthening
the family relationships in my life.

Through moving and breathing, we unblock all sorts of
residual constrictions—including feelings of pain that we
have not consciously acknowledged, sometimes for many
years. When this happens, the intimate connection with
those closest to you starts to shine with a new light, because you acquire a direct intimacy with these emotions
rather than avoid them.

Emily's story demonstrates what can occur when more
than one family member commits to practice, and then
shares the transformative benefits. This doesn't mean that
you can change the past or undo prior behavior, but it
does show that it's possible to honestly embrace the feelings and experiences that you share with your family
members. This happens by becoming wholly immersed
in life, including its sadness. You have to feel the life all
around you, as your breath, as your body, and in all relationship to others.

Working with Love

Unless you work in an isolated profession, your coworkers
share a great deal of your time. Often they are people you
know very little about—strangers, even. You might view
them within the context of the various positions they hold

within an organization, connected only by dotted lines and arrows explaining the functional and pragmatic relationship necessary to get the job done. If this is the case, then you're missing opportunities to relate intimately to real people.

The dynamics of the workplace can lead to stress and unhappiness that reverberate throughout other aspects of our lives. I will share with you my own deeply personal experience with this very issue.

For a period of some years, I'd forgotten to do my own practice. Maybe *forgotten* is the wrong word, but with all the other imperatives that seemed more important at the time—raising a family, making a living—I'd convinced myself that I just didn't have the time. This coincided with several stressful years of working in very high-level corporate telecommunications companies. I had a large staff, large responsibilities, and a large budget. The politics of internal and external competition were extremely demanding, if not nerve wracking. At times I felt I was being eaten up by a machine and was barely able to cope with the day-to-day cut and thrust. I was always reacting to challenges and getting through moment by moment instead of mastering my world.

Finally, the stress load began to show up in my poor health, emotional and physical, until I remembered one day to resume the practice. Observing how bad I was feeling, I was suddenly motivated to make room in my life for something that had once been at its core. My teachers had always said that the unavoidable motive of practice is suffering. When we observe our difficulties, we get the necessary insight to take practical action. One of my teachers would always say, "Everything is the truth, my restriction is the truth—and thank God for my restriction, because it has moved me to practice."

I was certainly moved to practice that year. So I did. And I was shocked at the result. I felt well again immediately! I became quiet and clear in mind. I was stunned that I had forgotten to do it for so long. The first thing I noticed in the office was that I was feeling good about everybody around me, even the people I'd had difficulty with in the days before—including my bosses, with whom I'd had some serious disagreements. I suddenly felt a friendly regard toward them. I began to eat my experience rather than letting my experience eat me. Aliveness seemed to be the senior principle of my body and breath, and my relationships with everybody. I found new and easier ways to deal with issues. I simply enjoyed being with people in this aliveness, and so we dealt with work problems with a lightness that hadn't been there before. I couldn't believe how effective the practice was. The power of this experience led me to want to make this available soon to everybody, everywhere.

When your relationship with a primary partner or spouse becomes the priority in your life, even more than work, then the juice of that relationship fuels all of your other activities. I found that the relationships at home with my wife and kids became a priority, became juicy, and stood on their own without being diminished by the stress I brought home from work. The flow at home fueled my passions at work. Things got really good that year, and

I've practiced ever since. The relationship with my wife became the priority of my life. It was like I remarried Robyn. I had married *her,* after all, not my corporation. The male-female relationship became the hub around which all other activities were ordered, and the juice of this relationship flowed into the rest of my life. When I began my practice again, the intimacy was extended to everyone. We renewed our vows! I promised myself to practice! I often joke now that couples should include a vow to do their daily practice of the Promise. But it's a serious joke. We became married to each other and not to our institutions, but our employers truly benefited from the positive energy we took to work.

In the big picture, all institutions of the world are there to serve and improve the quality of life. The secular is there to serve the sacred, which is the intimate relationship with our families and all others. When we forget this order of things and marry our work instead of our spouses, there is inevitable trouble as we take our eye off our intimate life as the very reason that we work.

What I came to see is that every person we share time with, be it at work or elsewhere, exists in relationship to us in a tangible way. The difference with our working lives is that we often see our work as an obligation and consequently dismiss the relationships as less important than those in our nonwork lives. Yet the life you live, as it is given to you, includes relationships in all forms. Whether they come in the guise of manager, cleaner, bus driver, receptionist, or school principal, your colleagues at work have relationships with you. You affect them, and they affect you. If a day at work involves a negative interaction with a coworker, this often causes anxiety and stress even when you are not at work. When relations are harmonious, though, it's a very different story. Sometimes you take to people you work with and come to see them as friends. But this is not always the case. Either way, the direct intimacy you experience as your moving body or breath allows you to accept and nurture others as the life that they are, not just their social identities or personalities. When you incorporate the principles of the Promise into your life and use the basis of intimacy as the foundation, all relationships improve.

Amy Hansen, whom you met in chapter 3, has found that using her practice in the context of her work as a physician has been a pathway to much greater fulfillment and happiness for herself as well as her patients. As a result, those she cares for have benefited as well:

The nature of the Promise has since spread to all areas of my life. I am a chronic pain doctor, and I include this into my time with my patients. It seems to me that the lack of true intimacy in the world today is leading to an increase in chronic pain, and so my goal is to work with those suffering from chronic pain by helping them reconnect to their true nature and the innate wisdom of their own bodies. I have found that increasing intimacy through breath and movement helps them feel better. I show them how to do the focused breathing that is part of the core practice, and it has helped.

Intimacy Within and Without

Recently, I was spending time in a beautiful part of the world where many varieties of plants abound. Walking among them, I noticed something quite wonderful. The lush papaya trees that were heavy with fruit grew not alone but in partnership. Where there was a fruit-bearing female plant, a male plant would be next to it, the two of them growing together silently in perfect harmony. It is a powerful example of the intrinsic knowledge in all life. There is no need for struggle or disharmony, because life actually knows what it is doing.

Look at a tree. We see a powerful trunk rooted deeply to stand erect. It is hard and upright; the eternal strength of life. When we get up to the foliage, we see that it is soft and succulent. Every leaf is so juicy and wide open. There the nutrients are received and collected for the health and well-being of all the trees. Their subtle chemistries are shared, transported by the wonder of life to ensure the continuity and improvement of all other trees. Without the foliage, the trunk would wither. Without the magnificent trunk, there would be no foliage. This is exactly how your wonder-full life is functioning. You have a masterful base and spine that support your soft crown and receptive front. All of life is strength receiving. This is the nature of reality; the natural state of all things. This is why we move and breathe to participate in what is natural.

It is now time to trust the life-giving force in yourself, as yourself, and participate in the profound union of all the life polarities that are clearly already given to you. What will happen is that in regaining your own sense of visceral and lived connection to breath and sex, an authentic sense of compassion and connection to all other organisms will arise. Becoming intimate with your reality—your own personal biology, no less—will have the flow-on effect of enhancing your innate sensitivity to all forms of life, and all forms of relationship, whether with people, plants, animals, or sun and moon and sky!

When you see that your breath is a gift from nature, it will become clear that you are part of a vast, complex network of life systems. Plants and animals, earth, water, fire, and air—the whole of Mother Earth—belong to the wonder of Nurturing Source Reality, and your birthright is to feel this sacred connection within every cell of your body, within every movement of your breath.

The Promise Practice will reignite your inner fire for your everyday life and intimate relationships with people, animals, plants, and the universe. The energy generated by the practice will begin to ebb and flow throughout your system, throughout your life, spreading out expansively like the branches of an enormous tree reaching up and out, embracing the experience of this life. Not as something manufactured or manipulated in any way, but as participation in the eternal and organic experience of your own breath and body. By extension, when we develop this natural relationship with ourselves, it will move into relationship with "others." It is not about making life into something it is not, but rather *feeling* more deeply the life that we have. Some aspects of the natural world will always feel less comfortable, like pain and grief, but we have avoided these at the vast expense of losing touch with our essence. Tangible experience of our own reality has been covered over and replaced with the desperate optimism of mere beliefs and the methods of hope that are cranked out to exploit the public suffering. Only through the embrace of all ordinary conditions can we grow, and move into the wonder that is us. In the depth of life that beats the heart and moves within you as breath and sex, you know the source of life. In the union of opposites, we know the Source of opposites and its nurturing power.

Your World, Welcome!

Just as the tree requires nothing extra to confirm its authenticity, neither do we. There need be no more seeking for what or who we are, because in our being that is expressed through breath and sex, we *are* the full-blown wonder of life. Our very own unique biology has for too long been denied as an inferior condition that should be overcome or transcended. Is it any wonder, then, that in our dismissal of our own, organic, natural processes—the living breath and sex—the same mistaken psychology has infiltrated the way we see our relationship with nature? We fearfully attempt to control and exploit our resource rather than receive it. In so doing, we are destroying our own ecosystems. Ultimately, the earth is not at risk, but we humans and other species are. No matter what happens, this great universe will restore its perfect systems with or without humans. These issues are not separate, and they hold great potency for the potential of healing that must occur in order to bring the natural balance of our physical world back into harmony. If we let ourselves feel our pain, others' pain, and the pain of the animal kingdom, we cooperate with pain and respond in practical ways.

CHAPTER 6

Pain Is Healing

Only through embracing all ordinary conditions can we grow, and move into the wonder that is us. Trusting in Nurturing Source allows you to explore the depth of life that beats as your own heart, and moves within you as breath at all times.

MOTHER NATURE IS NOTHING BUT A REGENERATIVE, nurturing, abundant continuity. Therefore, everything that is intrinsic to nature is also that—including sex and pain. Nature has one interest only: to regenerate, evolve, and improve life. Pain is a function of nurturing nature. It is the healing that ensures your maximum well-being and longevity. Inherent to the function of pain is its cessation as conditions change and improve. It demands change. It is literally a biochemical and energetic regeneration in the system. Your body is operating in extraordinary ways beyond scientific understanding, and you are in safe hands. So relax into and obey pain, allowing the changes it demands. If we did not have pain, we would not survive. *Take your hand out of the fire!* So the next time you feel pain, try to regard it as a friend and guide. Know that healing and change are occurring.

Relax into pain. But do so in cooperation with Mother Nature's caring hand. Where you experience chronic physical pain, move the affected or injured area in its natural elasticity with the breath, without causing further trauma. The therapeutic method is strength receiving, inhalation-exhalation through the whole body. The nurturing force then flows through you, removing the obstacles from your inner and outer pathways. It is unstoppable and dependable. Your Promise Practice facilitates this healing. Breathing with your legs rested above the trunk, as one part of the practice advises, is most restorative.

Pain is not the enemy. Even when it is chronic, it is still the healing. When you understand this, you may be able to endure it, knowing that pain is natural and is present for good reason. Know that life can cope with any amount of pain, and, when necessary, the body can even produce its own natural narcotics, or brain chemicals called endorphins (literally, "inner morphine"). The mind can relax from fearful reaction to pain, knowing that you are being healed, while carefully using modern pain management. If you feel exhausted, it's a message. Obey nature's intelligence. Rest. Soon life will restore you.

Finally, the ultimate healing by necessity is death. When your work in this world is complete, and the body is exhausted, you heal into death. It is like being in your mother's arms as she takes you home to the source of all. Everything is as it should be.

Conventional opinion would have us believe that pain

prevents us from moving forward in a positive way, and is consequently a restriction that needs to be removed. We are presented with a variety of methods that seek just to get rid of pain. In so doing, we deny its fundamental healing function. Some teachers suggest that pain is merely a habit that we dramatize—even a kind of phantom phenomenon that sort of follows you around. They point out that we get organized around this pain, behaving and choosing our relationships for its continuity, fearing it as if it were an entity, like a medieval devil. Their idea is that you can be free of pain by simply being conscious of it. Witness it only, they say, because getting involved with it creates further drama.

This is a valid idea worth considering. What I am saying, however, is that pain is real and has its function. Most of it has been caused by the generational denial of life, passed on through society. Pain is demanding that we change, and it must be acknowledged, embraced, and made use of, not feared. Doctrines have been made up by men who wanted nothing to do with birth, life, motherhood, and pain. Many have said that they felt life as utter misery, and they felt no choice but to drop everything about life.

I respect everyone's experiences, but I don't think that is a valid universal doctrine in a world of real details: relationships, sex, money, and diapers. They or their followers turned their experiences into worldwide teachings that deny the realities of pain, sex, life, and motherhood. I am saying that this aloofness is actually causing the pain that their methods are now trying to overcome. Witnessing your experience rather than embracing it turns everything into "other" by the mere fact that you are witnessing it instead of digesting it. The universal monastic method of renunciation has pervaded all of society's attitudes and behaviors and taken intimacy from humanity everywhere. What we need is intimate connection to life. It is only this that reduces the pain. The attempt to reside in awareness of negative patterns is now used in modern psychotherapy, or recognition therapy. As I said, it may be valid to recognize painful patterns, but what is most needed is a practical means for an intimate life. Instead of handing out meditation, mental health drugs, and philosophies, what we need is our life. Do these amidst the primary practice of intimate connection. Your Promise Practices of body, breath, and relationship will provide what you really need.

I maintain that the freedom the great Buddha speaks of is attained entirely in the other direction: not by avoiding "attachment" but in embracing breath, sex, and motherhood. I joke about this and say that he should have stayed with his wife in the palace and used his princely position to feed the people, to let the nurturing flow, instead of creating this dissociation for humanity. And what the Buddha actually said is up for debate anyway! My view is that the Buddha's liberation was absolute intimacy, absorption in every aspect of the natural life. The practices of awareness meditation dissociated from practices of intimacy arose as doctrinal practice hundreds of years later. Residing as the Witness only to all conditions is a basic template for many world teachings. For example, the Christian monastic life and the society it created, and many new age teachings of the West, are based on this ideal. Not getting involved with experience, the assumption goes, allows you to be free of any associated pain. This all-pervasive attempt has dissociated us from the natural state and exaggerated outbursts of aberrant human behavior—ironically, causing even more pain. Contrary to this method, the great ancient alternative is to take experience on in every aspect, to digest and embrace it, pleasurable and painful, and now it is real.

To be prepared to acknowledge pain brings awesome results. As with Gautama Buddha, usually only in times of suffering are we forced to stop and reflect on the conditions of our life. Painful experiences stop you in your tracks, tell you to pay attention, stand up, and evaluate your situation, and take the action required to get your life right. When life is moving in the direction that you want it to, you feel little impetus for reflection and, consequently, little motivation to move deeper into yourself. So pain is a gift. Yet we tend to view pain as something that needs to be opposed, fought against, and overcome. In the attempt to obliterate it, we become blind to the positive messages it conveys and the transformation that is possible through a personal experience of pain. A mother was telling me how exhausting it had been for her trying to overcome pain with the new age advice of finding her awareness principle residing as the witness in the midst of the bills and the washing and the growing pains of her little ones. Further, her self-esteem was diminished not only because she was in pain but also because she was unable to achieve what the teachers were telling her. A double whammy!

To be clear, the content of our troubled minds is created by a lack of intimacy. Think about it. What troubles your mind? In intimate connection, the mind is focused, alert, and peaceful. It is as simple as that. Meditation has been invented to free us from the content of our troubled mind by witnessing it instead of getting involved in it. Fair enough. Do that. But do it simply as an understanding, a refinement, in the midst of intimate practice. Detachment as a practice has dissociated humanity from our inherent connection to the natural state, to the body and all its relatedness. And please understand that the primary spiritual practice is intimacy. It cuts through your troubles like a hot knife through butter. Connection is the primary spiritual method by which we know ourselves, our life prior to and beyond the troubled mind. Troubles vanish. You will no longer need to attempt meditation as detachment; real meditation, *clarity of mind,* arises spontaneously and powerfully as you rest in your body, breath, relationship, and the Source of all arising conditions. We need to connect!

We can have a new relationship with pain, and know it as a sign of growth and healing. If you didn't experience pain, you would leave your hand in the fire, stay in harmful relationships and addictions of all kinds, and never be prompted to grow and change. Relaxing into pain allows you to move deeper into the nurturing field. Mothers tell me that the more they relaxed and cooperated with the pain of giving birth, the easier was the birth. Motherhood, pain, and love are inseparable and are the substance of reality. The natural flow of nurturing is the compassion so valued in world faiths as we take care of one another and ourselves in the pain that demands its own reduction. It is the mother's anguish over a vulnerable child or your love for a dying, defenseless parent. Being willing to feel pain takes us to love.

My teacher used to say, "Thank God for my pain, because it has enabled me to practice." He called it the "unavoidable motive to practice" that moves you to take the practical steps to enjoy your life.

By the gentleness of its daily discipline, your practice teaches you to participate in the natural intimacies that you have already been given. The resulting health alleviates your pain. The essential ingredient is not simply the breath but also your own intimate relationship *with* your breath and *with* life. This allows the healing power intrinsic to life to function most efficiently. We all breathe, certainly and essentially, but we usually forget all about our breathing. The daily practice of breathing and moving, as described in the later chapters of this book, will develop an intimacy with your breath and with your self. This intimate connection is the great healing. You are participating *with* your breath, consciously and compassionately, in the fullness of life itself. The result is regeneration and health: the goal of Mother Nature.

Take this story as an example. A friend of mine, a powerful young journalist, was describing vividly the sadness in her early life, her father's pain, and his abusiveness. His pain had been passed on to her as her own fundamental experience of life.

I remember watching my father threatening to kill my mother if she didn't get up off the floor. He was the reason she was there, because he had hit her so many times, I was surprised she could get up at all. I stood watching in shock, nine-year-old eyes struggling to compute. Over the years, there were more scenes of abuse and alcoholism, of asking my mother why she was crying, of feeling ashamed and scared, and of running away and coming back. One day, about five years later, my mother came to me and said, "I'm leaving. Do you want to come?"

We left with nothing and never went back. The experiences of my childhood caused me a lot of pain and passed on some seriously destructive ideas about relationships and intimacy. A string of relationships characterized by distrust, low self-esteem, and control were the inevitable aftershocks. I was never willing to allow myself to be vulnerable, for fear of more pain, nor could I see that men could be amazing people as friends and as lovers.

I tried to obliterate the pain from my childhood with sex, drugs, alcohol, exercise, meditation, and therapists, and, above all, by never getting intimately close to anyone. I let myself be bullied in countless aggressive Yoga classes. Although all of this allowed me to access the source of my pain, and to some extent fleetingly express it, such behavior never provided me with a means to acknowledge and dissolve that pain inside. After years of this not working, I decided that I had to find a way to heal beyond trying to obliterate or intellectualize. Through the practice of the Promise, I learned to move gently into the pain in my hips, or release the energy from my heart as I opened my chest to the sky. As a result of these subtle movements, I feel that things are shifting in me on several different levels: physically, emotionally, spiritually.

But it's deeper than that. I used to think that you always had to be strong, but now I see that it is stronger to be soft sometimes, to allow yourself to be vulnerable and open. I know that by lashing out, I only harm myself. When conflict occurs in my life now, I want to heal rather than fight. I believe more in people, in men, and in life. I am replacing aggression with forgiveness and compassion. It's not exactly easy, but it feels so much better. What is happening is beautiful, but intensely difficult to describe. It's not as though life is suddenly and magically perfect. What I am certain of, though, is that I feel stronger, more sure of myself, and quietly amazing.

Sadly, stories like this are everywhere, and we live in a culture that has accepted abuse as the norm. Its physical manifestation, like the case described, reflects the deeply embedded psychological, emotional pain that is hardwired into us, and in seeking to escape it, we often revert to ineffective temporary measures such as obsessive exercise, alcohol, meditation, or Prozac. Yet my friend's example shows that acknowledging and accepting pain—connecting honestly to your pain as a part of yourself—allows the discomfort to move through you, be released, and transform you.

In the midst of limitation, there is a natural progression of emotions, in this order: fear, anger, pain, grief, sadness, compassion, forgiveness. Each is real and is to be honored, not bypassed; each is to be engaged in sequence while also predicting the next stage of emotion. Pain caused by generational abuse is the transforming agent. It is not some phantom to be dissolved by somehow taking the position of mere awareness.

My journalist friend, in her courage, was able to forgive her father and be free of this obstructing emotion that had plagued her adult life. By acknowledging her anger, she could feel the pain beneath it. By being with that pain and knowing that it was natural and entirely valid in her life, she was able to let it do its healing work. It moved her to feel sadness and compassion for herself and everybody. She saw the shoddy deal that had been dished out to her father, too, and was able to see an overview of our dysfunctional society from the vantage point of her intimate connection to life.

Through the practice of the Promise, her daily intimacy with her own life, she was able to feel everything there is to feel and be free of the limiting patterns that had been passed through the generations. She regenerated. A literal new generation began for her; future generations and even the past generation were freed to meet their liberated daughter. What a service.

Mary's Story: The Ordinary Is Divine

Mary, a farmer in a remote part of Ireland, suffered from depression for many years. Her story shows how resilient and capable of healing we naturally are.

I have struggled with anxiety and depression for a lot of my adult life. I find it difficult to come to rest within myself. I first came across the Promise while watching a program on Body in Balance TV. Over my life, I had become very suspicious of teachers and gurus who claimed to have the monopoly on truth. How-

ever, Mark was different. He was genuinely calm, very human, and unusually modest for a teacher. The Promise seemed to be something that was practical and doable. So I started to practice, and now find that rest comes so easily and lovingly.

Mark talks a lot about intimacy with life, and when I finish my practice, which I often do outdoors, I find myself looking at the sky and saying to the universe, "I love you." It just seems the right thing to say. I feel held and cherished by something I can't describe but know is there. This is what intimacy with life feels like to me. Like the ordinary is divine and the Divine is ordinary. I don't have to look outside the nuts and bolts of my own life to experience the transcendent. Of course, the condition of anxiety and depression continues, and I would rather it didn't, but without it, I don't think I would have developed a seeking mind and never would have found the Promise. I also admit to having a somewhat distracted and flighty nature, which can be a challenge to a steady practice. But that's the beauty of the Promise. If you can breathe, you can do it. It is there waiting for you to claim it, and it is never the wrong time, and it is never too late.

Often people tell me that they feel embarrassed to admit they are in pain or depressed. They are urged to suppress their pain and remain functional rather than take time to let pain move through them at a natural pace. Hear me now! If you are sensitive to life, you *should* be in pain! It is often an appropriate, natural response to the chaotic circumstances of this world. Pain is a dynamic process of change and healing that needs to be *felt* in order for it to do its transformative work.

One day I would like to host a workshop titled "Be

Miserable and Stay Miserable, Then You Will Know Love!"
That's a joke, but a serious joke! Love is being willing to
look at life as it is, to accept all of life—including our pain.

In the context of the Promise Practice, it is necessary
to allow your heart and body to process pain naturally,
and be as gentle to yourself as possible. Remember that
you are always nurtured. Even in the darkest nights of
depression and despair, immense transformation is taking place.

Seeing pain as a friend, as a teacher, allows you to re-
frame its purpose. When you do this, it will soon become
clear that the intimacy you develop with less comfortable
aspects of life and experience opens up the opportunity
for intimacy with all ordinary conditions—especially, intimacy with others. I always say that "depressed" means
"deep rest." Let it do its nurturing work.

CHAPTER 7

Sex Is Never "Just Sex"

*Sex is a sacred and powerful act of union and inti-
macy. It deserves the utmost respect. Yet often we can't
even mention the word* sex *without implying something negative, sleazy. Dignity needs to be restored to
this word. We need to resurrect honor to male and
female union.*

THE SOURCE OF LIFE IS FELT AS THE BREATH. EACH
cycle of breath unites the strong masculine qualities of
the exhalation with the receptive, feminine qualities of
the inhalation. The whole body becomes permeated by its
male and female qualities; the blissful absorption of one
to another. The body loves its breath, and the inhalation
loves the exhalation.

From intimacy with all conditions—life and breath—
the human need for intimacy with "other" naturally
arises. Far from being a dangerous or destructive force,
sexuality is a powerful reflection of your human identity,
your innermost desires, beliefs, values, and self-esteem.
Establishing a loving, intimate relationship is a celebra-

tion of life, and when you honor this completely, sexuality becomes a joyous expression of love between partners.

Sex as an expression of love arises when two people are willing to meet each other with authenticity and openness. When you connect with another on this level, you transcend insecurity, falseness, and pain, and the strength and beauty that arise as a result reverberate through your life. When you are well loved, you offer love to those around you. It really is that simple.

Just as your heart pumps blood through your arteries and veins, your body expresses an instinctive desire for sexual pleasure and intimacy. If you could untangle yourself from all social conditioning and act from a level of pure physical instinct, you would discover little resistance to the manifestation and cultivation of this vital and most sacred energy.

For most people, however, the wholeness of this expression is enmeshed in social expectation and mental limitation. The spiritual denial of sex, the commercial distortion of sex, and the pornographic exaggeration of sex make up a wide spectrum of repression and dysfunction. The result is a lack of sensitivity and connection.

"Casual" Relationships and Separation

Our present rates of divorce and separation indicate that our ability to connect intimately with "other" has gone astray. Many readers will have experienced the sadness that comes with the end of an intimate relationship, and the residual issues of fear and mistrust that often result from this loss. People often struggle to maintain the depth of connection and chemistry that initiated the relationship, and so they end up feeling estranged from each other. The quest to regain our ability to love freely can sometimes seem futile.

This hasn't been helped by the current climate, which presents sex as a saleable commodity rather than a sacred and powerful act of union and intimacy. Nor has it been helped by the popular endorsement of "casual sex" relationships.

How is it possible to find intimate connection with another, when so many messages tell us that sex is so often "just sex"? Even in this popularized saying, we are devaluing the powerful energy that is transferred between two people in the act of sex, and denying ourselves ultimate pleasure and fulfillment.

Frequently I hear from women who feel that the consensus among men today is that they want to have sex, but simply don't want to commit to ongoing intimacy and love. These poor men miss out on real sex, the sublime feeling of utter male-female union. They empty themselves in mere fleshly stimulation. It is like masturbating in the woman. They do not learn to gather her subtle energies in the safety of intimacy, and this is devastating for women too. These stories are reflected in many popular stories; for instance, the hit TV series *Sex and the City* made such narratives famous. Still, each of the women in that show—and all the women who speak to me of such things—continue to seek out that special connection. (Even Samantha Jones, the promiscuous character who reveled in treating her male lovers with the same dispatch as any stereotypical Don Juan, settled into her most permanent and apparently satisfying relationship after a brush with cancer.)

Intimacy is not a casual matter or a casual affair. The very word implies a connection beneath the surface of things; its original meaning was "most inward or deep seated." It is an opportunity to participate in the life of another. By doing so, you participate positively with the powerful, regenerative function of nature.

And even if, at the moment, you are not in a relationship with another person, you are in a relationship nevertheless. That relationship is with yourself. With your body. With your breath. By cultivating that primary intimacy with yourself, you will cultivate intimacy with others.

This is the core principle of the Promise. The practice of breath and body movement, of strength receiving, exhalation and inhalation, done every day for a few minutes, will awaken all the intimacy you need in order to engage in a loving relationship with another.

I promise you: you can have this.

Martina's Story:
Strength and Receptivity

A scholarly friend from Byron Bay in Australia, Martina Duel, describes the tangible connection of exhalation and inhalation, or strength receiving, with the union of her own male and female characteristics:

I had a profound learning from the Promise seminar this weekend. After the morning session on the first day, I felt "weird," but not unpleasantly so. This continued all weekend, until by lunchtime on the second day, I figured out what I was feeling. I was experiencing, maybe for the first time ever, strength and receptivity at the same time!

For the past decade, I have been exploring masculine and feminine energy, in myself, in relation to others, and in existence, but I was uncomfortable. When "in my masculine," and getting things done, I felt too aggressive, single focused, and inflexible. Yet "in my feminine," I was a pushover! I had poor boundaries and was far too accommodating of others' desires. I had come to distrust both parts of myself, and was therefore quite stuck and cautious in many ways.

What I feel now is how very intimately these energies work together, and that I can be both simultaneously, instead of swinging neurotically between the two. The key to this was discovering my inhalation to be a gift, one I had only to receive. This opened up a receptive capacity in me as I experienced a true gift with no strings attached, perhaps for the first time in my life!

I feel very excited about living my life with the strength to support my feminine wisdom and love, and with receptivity and flexibility informing my strength of being and doing. I have already made decisions to change in areas I had been stuck in through not trusting my old ways of moving and being in the world. I will let you know how this unfolds.

What you must understand is that intimacy is the greatest aphrodisiac, and without it, the physical act of sex does not measure up. Our understanding of sex has been perverted by pornography culture, presenting the idea that sex is a type of performance or show, and taking no account of the primal energy that is exchanged between two people. Those who have been in a committed partnership come to realize that sex with deep and sincere affection is the most extraordinary human experience. It is something that simply cannot be achieved in the flippant throes of a one-night stand or even an illicit fling—these kinds of scenarios make light of the deep energy exchange that goes on during sex.

More often than not, women are the ones who feel most hurt by these events, in part perhaps because their bodies have produced potent binding chemicals that send signals to unite with the sexual partner on an ongoing basis. It's a bad deal for men, though, because pleasure in life comes from the honest receptivity to the feminine, not from controlling the feminine. This translates as receptivity to the natural state, not the control of the natural state.

What is required is a readjustment of the attitude we hold toward sex and gender roles. The misconception about male and female roles in the act of sex is a significant part of this problem, one that often leads to dissatisfaction in both men and women. Fulfillment of the male is not in the ending of his desire. Man's pleasure is actually in the pleasure of the feminine. When the power of the feminine is joined with the power of the masculine, something extraordinary happens. Such an accord or marriage makes a potent entity of the relationship itself, with no requirement for artificial "sexiness" or performance—just real feeling.

Yet this extraordinary something is really quite ordinary, because it is the natural state; the process of nature. This most fundamental force of life is happening through you, and assures the survival of our species. If you do not participate in this essential force, you live as if all your other options, including career, religion, sports, even the arts, are more vital than intimate partnership. The power of mutuality inherent in intimate relationship is stronger than any individual. You could also substitute the word *peace,* because you will enjoy the peace and power of your individual life in its vast integration with everything *and* enjoy life's movement to the opposite. One does not exclude the other; instead, one *allows* the other.

The Power of Stillness: An Intimate Exercise

Personal autonomy and partnership go hand in glove. Here is a short but powerful exercise that you can do anytime with your partner. Turn off the phone and TV and find a comfortable spot on the bed or floor. Lie next to your partner in the stillness of the moment. Rest in the feeling of your stillness and the stillness of the whole of life. After a short while, turn to each other and let the energy of life move between you. (You can even visualize this energy as interlocking lines of light and power, as in those marvelous paintings by Alex Grey showing the interplay of anatomical and spiritual forces in the subtle body. Or the beautiful lines of light in the healing scene in the movie *Avatar*.) Soon you are connecting with the powerful force that moves naturally from stillness. You may touch each other lightly at first and eventually move to a full frontal embrace.

An old song I'd heard in New Zealand goes, "There appears to be motion, but motion is still / The ocean is silent, and yet there's a thrill."

The practice of the Promise is the simple participation in life's movement of body, breath, senses, sound, and sex; from stillness and back to stillness.

If you can admit to your lover that you are more powerful *with* him or her than you are on your own, and this confession is felt and expressed mutually, that's a profoundly liberating event. You will discover a broad river of feeling flowing between you—as wide and deep as the immeasurable movement of life. This is a vulnerable place to be, and often we are afraid to go there. You may think that you'll be safer on your own without risking rejection, because whatever you find in union with another might someday be taken away. But this vulnerability itself is powerful, because it is true.

So if you find someone who can be this vulnerable with you, don't let that person go. You will enjoy your life together more than you will your lives alone. And I don't mean only the sexual aspect of mutuality but also the entire relationship. The mutual accord and enjoyment between equal partners grows when each is grateful to the other for what the union creates. The sexual union expresses this quality in a powerful way in the context of the whole.

Ana's Story: Passionate and Tender, Easy and Fun

Once when I was teaching a workshop in Manhattan sponsored by a large learning center known as the Omega Institute for Holistic Studies, I had a long conversation with its program director. Ana Sanjuan had a background in organizational development and a passion for holistic health. (She now works as a marketing consultant and coach.) In the course of our discussion, Ana revealed that her goal was to master certain spiritual practices. But with a couple of very young children at home, plus her demanding job at Omega, she had little time to accomplish everything, including a daily physical practice. I asked her if she would let me show her a simple practice that she could do in seven to ten minutes a day.

She agreed, and we stepped into one of the banquet rooms that were being cleared out for the next session. There, with workers milling around, I showed her the basic steps of the Promise, which I wrote down for her on a yellow legal pad. "If you'll promise me that you'll do this every day for three months," I said, "I promise you it will change your life." I didn't see Ana until the following year, when I came to the Omega campus in upstate New York to teach another workshop. That's when she made a fascinating revelation:

At the time, my husband and I had been really hauling butt—spending so much time working at our jobs and caring for our two toddlers that we virtually had to schedule time to spend together. It shouldn't have surprised me that my libido was sinking to new lows, and I didn't have time for long exercise classes to get my energy level back up. So when I started doing the Promise, it was just what I needed: seven minutes a day that made me feel refreshed and energized. Each day for three or four weeks, I would do this simple series, and once I promised to do a few minutes a day, it wasn't that hard. I started to feel the effects of quieting the mind. I have a great library of spiritual books, and I love to read them, but I never seemed to have time. So I would decide to pick up a spiritual book and read it for ten minutes. That had an effect on the rest of the day.

I subsequently went through a few weeks when I was all over the place and had a hard time focusing. I was feeling ornery and angry—and then I realized that I hadn't been doing my practice. I discovered that when I start my day with the Practice, I have a substantially different level of energy, so I went back to doing my Seven-Minute Wonder. Then one evening, I looked at my husband in the kitchen and stopped in my tracks. He looked so delicious. Spontaneously, I reached out and kissed him. It felt like the first time. I trembled, and he noticed. We both said, "Wow."

And from then on, it was different; I would drive home looking forward to the part of the night where our kids were tucked

away and we could be alone. Our sex was passionate and ten-
der, easy and fun. And when you are having a good, regular sex
life, everything is better: your communication, your social life,
the chores. The stress of kids and careers takes second place,
because you've regained your core; your union with your mate.

When that first happened with my husband, though, I didn't
immediately connect the surge in my libido to the Promise. In
the past year, I'd been exposed to so many teachers and healers
at Omega! I sat with John of God [a Brazilian healer and me-
dium] when he was there, and sat in on workshops with other
energy healers; my mother was even using the practice of ener-
gizing water, and I didn't know if one of those practices might
have triggered this surge. So I decided to experiment. I realized
that when I stopped doing the Promise, I could feel my sexual
energy level receding. And when I started the practice again, my
libido was reanimated.

My main concern when teaching Ana the Promise was
that she seemed obsessed with pushing herself to master
her spiritual practice, which included meditation. I sensed
that her seeking was leaving her feeling inadequate in her
day-to-day life. I told her that she was already a master.
She had "mastered" motherhood, the greatest mastery of
them all. I hadn't made a big deal out of how the practice
can improve physical intimacy, and may not have mentioned it at all. Our conversation was more about not trying to seek something outside of yourself, but to discover
what already exists within you.

When I ran into Ana that second time, she said, "Hey,
I have something to ask you!" After describing what had

been happening with her sex life, she asked, "Is this re-lated?" And, of course, it was.

"Hot damn!" she said. "You never told me." So we had a good laugh over that.

We tend to think of sex as something extra, like the cherry on the sundae. If you have rewarding work to do, enough money for your needs, a good relationship, family, a spiritual life—then, oh yeah, some sex would be nice. But it's just the other way around. As Ana put it later:

When sex is working, everything else is in alignment: you're communicating, being more compassionate, more relaxed and calm, and you feel fulfilled. It's not the sex itself so much as the rest of the day and the rest of the week. The reason you started a family was because you were turned on to each other and felt good being together, and that feeling can become obscured. So that was not planned; I didn't know that was going to happen, but I was very pleased. The Promise enriches other practices I do. The Promise kicked everything back into place.

Once you establish this depth, you may not always feel it continuously. You may find obstructions along the path. But the more you practice the Promise, especially with your partner, the more likely you'll be to continue feeling intimate.

The biggest drawback to the various mythologies sur-rounding masculine and feminine identities is that they overshadow the inherent need for the union of the male and female polarities within our system. The stereotypes that men are strong and women receptive are alienating for both genders, and reduce what should be a mutual collaboration—meeting each other from a place of authenticity—into a power play. The union of the masculine and feminine already occurs in each of us, regardless of gender. It is not a matter of women behaving more like men, or men like women, for what we call male and female aspects manifest differently and uniquely in each person. As a consequence, it is vital that sexual union be expressive of these qualities; otherwise we are doing little more than creating pain by playing out the dramatization of the social mind. Reclaiming and restoring the dignity to sex means throwing away a whole range of misconceptions and tortured beliefs, which may require conscious unraveling after years of negative experiences.

Victoria's Story: Intimacy with Self

Throughout my life, sexuality was either instant gratification, like a piece of chocolate cake, or dirty and hidden, like my being sexually abused when I was a child. From the Barbie doll into which I wished my body would take shape, to the relationships in soap operas and Hollywood movies that fed me lies, the male vision of sexuality was all around me. I used sex as a way to control life, until one Saturday night when I was sixteen. I was raped, and it made me feel dirty instead of angry. Like many women in that situation, I really believed that it was my fault that I was raped, because I had been promiscuous. I hated myself, and hated my sexuality.

It is so conflicting to grow up in this country where the media portray this male vision of sex, and yet if a woman really embraces her sexuality, she is a slut. So I viewed my sexual options as either being in a monogamous relationship—maybe acting out what we saw on porno films to try to spice up our sex life—or years of being single and having one-night stands. Either way, I bonded superficially with sex so that I could hide the real me, which I was convinced no one would love. The one-night stands usually involved large amounts of alcohol. In my drunken state, I would be able to connect intimately, but when I was sober, I was too afraid to open up. I was a prisoner within my own sexuality and suffered because of it.

My late twenties and early thirties became a time of sexual experimentation. As I acted out my suppressed anger, I kept flogging myself and hating myself even more. And then, in my midthirties, I shunned my sexuality and was basically celibate, completely disconnected from my true nature.

Then I found an exercise practice that I thought could work. At first I used it just like I had used sex. If I could look like the teacher and do the most advanced pretzel-shaped pose, maybe I would be better. However, I couldn't do it, and this made me even more upset with myself. I would then crash into despair and stop practicing for periods of time. As my last long-term relationship crashed and burned, so did this old practice.

Luckily, something had seeped in and made a subtle, irreversible change. I had found a connection with my own heart. I started to cultivate a relationship with myself through my own practice. I started to listen to myself, take care of myself, and *eventually really love myself. Through attention to the body and, therefore, the breath, I became more intimate with myself. It started in my practice and then spread to all aspects of my life.*

I still desire a partner to share my life with, but I want an intimate relationship with myself even more. I can get hung up on the desire for partnership, but I'm lucky because I have learned to keep returning to my practice, and to intimacy with myself. This has changed my relationships. I am currently starting a new one, and instead of bringing in the past and being fearful of the vulnerability, I am enjoying it. I am sharing my intimate heart. I am not acting out with expectations based on fear. I am sharing "lovesex," not "fearsex."

As Victoria's experience shows, embodying generations of sexual negativity can be painful and difficult to work through. While men and women may have different ideas about what intimacy entails, it is up to individuals and couples to negotiate that for themselves rather than play the appropriate roles laid out for them. The best relationship consists of an association of autonomous individuals who freely choose to be with each other. That doesn't mean promiscuity or sex for personal gratification but simply as an expression of love and a desire for mutuality with your intimate other. The power of life is in the sexual union. Life energy moves through you in this form, for this purpose. We are designed for love and intimacy even if we might struggle to admit it! We are built as these perfectly upright, embracing creatures. The fronts of our bodies are open and soft, and our skin is a feeling mechanism.

Everything that exists within the natural world is involved in a relationship of interdependency. Our survival depends on our unending embrace of and connection to each other. When two people say to each other, "You are my power," the current of life is free to flow endlessly between them. Sexual empowerment lies in getting in touch with your body and discovering this in your own way. By acknowledging your mutuality with each other and recognizing the source of your peace and power, you can begin to move in an infinitely positive and healing direction.

God and Sex: Now You Get Both

While we can draw much guidance and inspiration from religious and spiritual texts, we should not depersonalize our loving of each other in favor of an abstract notion of universal love, or love for one's God. You, and everyone in your life, are as much a part of the universe and as much a manifestation of God as the oceans, trees, space, and sky. Only through our intimate embrace of each other can divine love genuinely be known. And when we place value and dignity on the sexual union—the most potent connection we can have with another being—we connect directly to the source of life. This is why it is said in the traditions that a man and a woman can bring each other to God.

This sublimity is predicated on an actual body and breath practice and sensitivities that the Promise provides. To be inspired by the great literature or the new age ideas of "sacred sex" and imported notions of Indian Tantra without learning a practical means is fruitless. (Tantra is the vast tradition of the individual's union with the universe via all natural relationships. It forms the shamanic origin of all religion. The Promise Practice is the central pillar of making this tradition come alive today.) As I have said, beautiful ideas without the means to realize them can only makes matters worse. The good news is that if you have been inspired, the Promise offers you a tangible way to do something about it.

While spiritual texts and concepts have inspirational value, they have no practical use unless you can integrate them with your primary connection to your body, breath, and inherent perfection. Various religious tools—prayers, texts, mantras—can be used to acknowledge intimacy, but they become most powerful only when they are free of a limited belief system. In the religious denial of intimacy and sex, the guilt that many traditions associate with sexual pleasure has driven a wedge between our natural bodily desires and our innate life source. This primal and sacred union between humans has been framed as a lesser act—indeed, one that leads *away* from spiritual experience. Sex has been positioned as a lowly desire that must be transcended in order to achieve enlightenment or get closer to the Divine. Some traditions treat sex as a necessary evil that is allowed only to procreate children. Even those that acknowledge the need for sex to bind a couple in love often live in the shadow of the Apostle Paul's biblical exhortation to widows and the unmarried: "If they cannot exercise self-control, they should marry.

For it is better to marry than to burn with passion"(1 Corinthians 7:9). These teachings have filtered down over the centuries and permeated all aspects of our culture, causing great harm. The denial of our innate need for bodily connection has bred the false ideas that your body, flesh, heartbeat, breath, and capacity for sexual pleasure are polar opposites of godliness or spirituality.

Respect for yourself, your body, and the preciousness of sex supports a social order based on love and nurturing instead of control and denial. Denying sex only causes serious pain and dysfunction, as we have seen from the practice of celibacy, for example. When you hold your breath for too long, you can't help but gasp for air when you inhale. In the same way, "holding in" sex has only intensified its erotic appeal, with the result that it may manifest in damaging and pathological ways across the religious spectrum. Celibacy is not a measure of strength but an indication of confusion—namely, the mistaken belief that sexual practice somehow conflicts with profound levels of spiritual realization.

For those whose lives are aligned closely with a religious practice, the presentation of sexual abstinence as a spiritual ideal can be a difficult concept to integrate—and a philosophy that is nearly impossible to attain. The most common result is a guilt-engendered attempt to compartmentalize life. Enjoying your body, having sex, and raising a family are often seen as lesser pursuits than renouncing sex and family in favor of seeking higher spiritual realization. Paradoxically, this viewpoint has created a way of life that actually obstructs God realization or Buddhahood, and has introduced a kind of hierarchy in which the regular householder life is deemed of less value than the calling to be a priest, monk, or nun, whether of a Western or Eastern order. Before Buddhism arose about 2,500 years ago, there was no concept in the East of renunciation or celibacy as a spiritual ideal. In fact, the ancients considered an intimate family life the most auspicious circumstance for a spiritual life, one in which each and every individual was worthy of utter respect. Even in Christianity, the tradition of celibacy for priests, monks, and religious women did not come into common use until around a thousand years ago, and then largely to keep church land from being divided among the offspring.

When it comes to sex, women seem to have gotten an especially raw deal, a lose-lose situation in which they are positioned as either guardians of virtue or seductive temptresses. Female sexuality is represented as a potentially dangerous, corrupting force that must be contained; within the family realm, sex is valued only for its reproductive capacities, not for how its pleasure makes women feel complete! Even if you are not religious, you may find that these paradigms have become etched in your social psyche, continuing to color your experience of sex and intimacy.

Nor is this attitude toward sex limited to the Western monotheistic traditions. After his enlightenment, the Buddha broke with the conventions of his time and place by openly teaching men and women of different castes. And yet he was still concerned about having women within his inner circle, because he thought they would be a distraction to his monks! He taught love and compassion but didn't say much about sexual intimacy. (One of his senior disciples eventually convinced the Buddha otherwise, and he did found an order of Buddhist nuns—led by the woman who had been his wife when he left on his journey to discover the solution to human suffering.) The Indian tradition has also glorified wandering holy men who live celibate lives that supposedly mark them as "holier than thou."

The idea that withdrawing your attention from physical intimacy with another person will somehow free up energy to focus on spiritual devotion or love of God is misguided at best. Love is always an intimate affair. Intimate relationships are the vehicle by which we experience and express our love. Attempting to depersonalize your loving by placing it in a larger context, such as universal love of humanity, or love for God, will only succeed in watering it down. And please discard the absurd premise that you can have God *or* sex, but not both. It's simply not true. Sex and spirituality are one and the same and cannot be dissociated. I have been stunned to hear young sophisticates assume that it must be one or the other, and then struggle with the consequences. This uninspected assumption is still with us, and it has reduced sexuality among young people to an act that is either very casual and unsatisfying ("friends with benefits") or a danger to life and health because of the rise of sexually transmitted diseases. It is time for a change, time for an education, because now you can indeed have both God and sex.

When you value and respect the sexual union, you

connect to the source of life. The infinite flow of life energy springs from the source that has formed your life as a system of opposites in union. It is a literal flow of feeling through the whole body, like a great river that nurtures and cleanses you, broad and dependable—heaven on earth. This is a promise.

CHAPTER 8

The Union of Opposites

Sex, the utter union of male and female, created your father and your mother, whose intimacy, in turn, created you. Sex is not an obstruction to knowing our Source but the very means of knowing it.

THE PROMISE PRACTICE DRAWS ITS STRENGTH FROM one of the oldest principles in human consciousness: participation in the union of all opposites. When you combine left and right, front and back, above and below, inhalation and exhalation, strength and receptivity, male and female, within and without, spirit and form—when you have all those opposites connected, the power of polarity generates enormous potential, like the electrical energy that surges between the positive and negative poles of a battery.

One reason people say that opposites attract is that each one complements the other, and together they are much stronger than the sum of their parts. The union of opposites allows the power of spirit to take material form in its ultimate expression.

Participation in the union of opposites reveals the source of all opposites, which is the heart. The heart is the ultimate power and presence of reality that appears as everything. All opposites originate at and join in the heart, and from there they flow everywhere.

The First Cell of Life

Before we can continue to discuss the union of opposites, we need to say a few words about the heart itself.

In the ancient world, the spiritual heart, known as the *hrid,* was considered to be the first cell of life to be formed through the perfect union of male and female. The word *hrid* means both to give (*Hr*) and receive (*Dh*). This simultaneous union represents the power of life, the power of sex, and the complete union and function of male and female.

By a process similar to the biological activity known as cell division, the heart rapidly divides and multiplies to become the whole body. In that sense, the heart *is* the whole body and all its function and relatedness. From the *hrid,* or heart, the whole body blooms in all its polarities, including its internal male-female polarities, which manifest as left and right, above and below, base and crown, front and back, strength and receptiveness, giving and receiving, and within and without.

The practice of the Promise is your participation in all the opposites encompassed by the heart—particularly as inhalation and exhalation, and strength that is receptive.

This is the key to sex, love, and intimacy.

It is the means—the *practical* means—to feel and participate in the natural state, the mysterious power and intelligence of life that is you and all your relatedness to the natural universe.

When you practice the Promise, you will feel a sense of *belonging* to life. This *is* the natural state. You *do* belong to life. You are as authentic to life as the sun or moon or a great tree or flowers that bloom.

Erotic Intimacy

In the ancient world of India, the soul's relationship with God was expressed by the image of an illicit love affair between a human incarnation of God and a beautiful young woman. Krishna, an incarnation of the great god Vishnu, was already married—indeed, he had eight official wives! But according to the ancient texts, Krishna spent much of his youth in the company of young cowherd girls, called *gopis,* whom he entertained by playing the flute.

While Krishna was married, he carried on an affair with one of these gopis, whose name was Radha. They were besotted with each other. This affair has been celebrated for centuries in Indian myth and poetry as a metaphor for the soul's relationship with the Divine. The erotic intimacy between Krishna and Radha, which was secret (and therefore seen as illicit), came to stand for the powerful attraction of the soul to God.

What the ancient metaphor is really saying is that

your relationship with Source Reality is extremely private, deeply personal, and utterly passionate. I want *you* to be besotted with Source Reality, to love your life as passionately as you would a secret lover. And I'm promising you that you can.

By doing the Promise, participating in the union of opposites on a daily basis, you will tap into your primary intimacy (it's already there, remember; no need to go seeking it). Like working a muscle, this intimacy will strengthen. It will then extend to others very naturally. If you are not in a relationship and wish to be in one, the Promise will make you more receptive and open to finding a compatible mate. And if you are in a relationship, you will feel more passionate toward your spouse or partner.

This is especially true if your partner joins you in the practice. When you practice together, you support each other and share the experience. This in itself is wonderful. But even better is the intensity of passion that arises. There are two of you, each participating in the intimacy of body movement and breath, and sharing that intimacy with each other. I promise you, it gives you a passionate union that is quite unknown, quite different from our conventional view of relationship and marriage. It is discreet, passionate, and very private. It gives you what you are yearning for often in spiritual or religious seeking. It is the realistic enactment of these sublime states and the proposed relationship with God described in the abstract.

Your practice can also help to restore intimacy. You may have had the experience of being in a relationship that has lost the passion that used to animate it and make it so much fun. Then you meet someone else and feel the spark that you used to feel with your partner. In most cases, it's a mistake to end your current relationship to take up with someone else, because unless you learn how to generate and maintain intimacy, the same distance and dullness will eventually set in. Then you'll have to find *another* someone else to restore the spark—leading to an endless string of unsatisfying relationships.

Instead you need to re-create that spark of intimate connection with your current partner. If that's not possible, and he or she won't play with you, then the honorable thing to do is to end the relationship as graciously as you can, in gratitude for all it has given. Before you do anything else, though, please spend a significant amount of time with your body and breath practice. It will work its magic for you.

The union of opposites is present in symbolic form in all the great traditions. It is wondrous to me that the Jewish Star of David and the Indian *Sri Yantra* appeared in the ancient world in utterly different regions and cultures, and at different times, yet they are quite similar: two overlaid triangles, one pointing up and one pointing down, reflecting the ancient saying, "As above, so below."

The same concept is embodied in the familiar East Asian symbol known as yin and yang. The Tibetans call it *yab-yum,* or "father-mother," the depiction of a male bodhisattva and his female consort in intimate sexual embrace. The bodhisattva embodies the ancient Buddhist

ideal of one who willingly postpones his or her final enlightenment until all beings are saved. This highlights the
understanding that compassion, the flow of Life's nurturing force in relationship, is more the point than even the
ideal of enlightenment. In this equation, the male principle is called by a term signifying "skillful means," and
the female principle by a word meaning "wisdom." (In the
Hebrew Bible, as well as in its later Greek translation, the
words for *wisdom* and *spirit* are both feminine in gender.)

The magnetism at the heart of the Radha-Krishna
romance is the union of opposite polarities in the form
of male and female. This whole-hearted love is erotic in
the most positive sense of the word. It is eros love, the
esoteric mysticism of the individual's union with God.

By your participation in, and your intimacy with, the
union of opposites, you learn to enjoy your deeply passionate relationship with Nurturing Source Reality. And
be aware that you must experience this *within yourself*
before you can experience it with another person. This is
the purpose of the daily practice that I will teach you in
the second half of this book.

Just as above with below, exhalation with inhalation,
you will find that strength with receptivity enacts this
mystical love affair with life.

Going to Love

Love is not sex. Yet human beings can feel and express
their intrinsic sense of union and shared life through

sexual intimacy. Love is all about relating to another at a level that approaches identifying with that person. And because our bodies have soft, feeling skin, and strong, upright spines, we can express that love sexually.

Love is also personal—it is the appreciation of an actual person. "Love your neighbor as yourself" is more than just a pious axiom; it is the essence of the human regard of one to another.

The imposition of ideas of "higher love" or "all-pervading consciousness" or "the ground of being" onto love depersonalizes human love and grossly distorts the role of sex within love. This deification of higher love is merely a variation on the old Manichaean belief that the spirit is good and the body is evil. That fallacy, dating back to third-century Persia, has insinuated itself over several thousand years into both Eastern and Western systems of religion and spirituality, including new age spirituality, with the result being either the degradation of sex by denying it, or the exaggeration of sex by separating it from love.

My teacher used to say, "Always yield to temptation." By this, he meant that one should refine and master pleasure, which is ultimately the subtle elixir of intimate life. Following our natural inclinations leads to the genuine intimacy that lies at the heart of love.

But the world's religions have all incorporated the idea of mastering your desires—by which they mean *suppressing* them. However, sex is too natural and powerful an instinct to be suppressed. Trying to suppress sex is like trying to suppress the breath; you just end up suffocating. Or it's like going on a starvation diet: you may lose weight, but you can become quite ill, and in extreme cases, people die from anorexia.

The imposition of celibacy on religious men in particular has had devastating effects on Western society, as we have seen. Over and over again, good and powerful men with high office and responsibility are brought to their knees through sexual misadventure. They simply cannot feel what they know in their hearts is a sublime human potential. It comes out as reckless affairs, naïve or sometimes even criminally abusive behavior in both secular life and religious institutions. I feel compassion for the abused as well as the abuser. Their lives have been damaged by misguided teachings. It's significant that the highest incidence of sexual crimes and misconduct in religious orders is among those on whom celibacy has been forced, or those who teach their congregations to be celibate as an ideal. This includes Roman Catholic clergy and orthodox Eastern gurus—male and female.

The notion that the denial of sex is the means to religious realization has it exactly backward. Sex is itself a *means* for realization. Many popular new age teachers, who are sincere and personally charming, write and speak in ways that can be inspiring. Yet they don't offer any practices or teachings that address the natural need for sexual intimacy that we all feel. They advise their followers to "go within," as if that were enough, but they don't deal with the need for intimate physical connection with another flesh-and-blood human being.

Reaching for God, or "the All-Pervading," without a physical practice that engages your sexuality diminishes the value of real personal love, regard, and touch. When you love the person in front of you for who and what he or she is, you can no longer tell the difference between your partner and the rest of existence. But when you go about it in reverse, trying to get to God by denying sex, it just doesn't work.

John Patrick: From Celibacy to Intimacy

When I first met John Patrick, he was living an austere life as a celibate monk in Santa Barbara, California. Years before that, as John Patrick Sullivan, he had been an All-American Hall of Fame middle linebacker at the University of Illinois and went on to play in the National Football League. His pro career was cut short in part by injuries but also, by his own admission, because of his high-life partying off the field. Forced to retire from the great game while only in his midtwenties, he said he felt dumped off at the parking lot, used up like a Vietnam veteran—no longer useful with his overtrained, overstrained body, with muscle bulk and strength that restricted his sensitivities to life. Dissatisfied with the world of name and fame, he began to search in the world of spirituality and religion. When we go to one extreme, we usually feel compelled to go to the other. But neither works.

When we met, John had pictures of the great Indian saint Sri Ramana Maharshi and other gurus on his wall, and he was practicing the essence of Vedantic teachings. Central to these teachings is the concept of nonduality, meaning that, ideally, there is no separation between you and the rest of creation: "all is One."

The irony is that to achieve the nondual state of awareness, you stand back and remove yourself as much as possible from the hurly-burly of everyday life. Instead of mixing it up, you learn to observe everything as a "witness." That may sound appealing, because it promises a level of serenity, but it can take you away from your own connection to ordinary reality.

In John's case, it included a vow of celibacy. He saw this as a way of countering the profligate life he had been carrying on as a football star. We had a couple of conversations, during which a more basic truth about his life emerged. Amid all the life options and Vedanta and everything else, what John really wanted was some good sex! But it wasn't wild, promiscuous sex he wanted. It was an intimate relationship with one person. I asked simply, "John! Where is your woman?" He told me later, in reference to his self-imposed celibacy, "I had to admit you were right, and that afternoon I phoned my future wife."

I didn't say to John, "Go out and pick up a chick." I suggested instead that he practice direct intimacy with his own reality—strength that is receiving. In a workshop I was leading, I taught him the Promise. He began to practice, moving and breathing for a few minutes every morning, and lo and behold, his capability of becoming receptive to the feminine opposite emerged suddenly. He met a woman who had been at the workshop, and they started dating. Before long, they had married and started a family.

Sometime later, I asked John if anything I'd been saying about opening up to the feminine sounded off base.

"No, you're right," he said. "The feminine was really what linked me back into the Source. The nondual conception that I was looking for in the monastery was actually right there in the merging of the divine feminine. That's what connected me to being present—and that entails also being in a relationship."

"We could, of course, delete the word *divine,*" I replied, "and just say *the feminine,* as it is manifested as the ordinary reality—your woman, in the flesh."

"The flesh and bones," he said, "with kids and family and the whole thing."

"The ordinary reality has arrived," I added.

"Yes, ordinary," John said.

"Nurturing Source appears," I said, "as this extreme intelligence that is the skin, the breath, the sex, the mother, the father, the child, the flowers growing in the fields. All ordinary conditions uniquely manifest as each individual, not to be suppressed or destroyed for the idea of some higher place somewhere else."

The more beguiling the religious text or teaching is, the more it dissociates you from this ordinary reality. Because John had a devotion to Ramana Maharshi, I felt it was important to remind him that Ramana's was a unique experience. As a young boy living in the southernmost part of India, Ramana spontaneously fell into a kind of coma. He emerged from that experience with a high level of realization. A rare and extraordinary event like this can ignite and fuel our desire for "enlightenment." We go seeking, hoping for a similar experience. If the utterances of a spontaneously realized saint are then turned into standardized text, we have an additional problem: we are reading words that may describe a state of bliss, but they do not offer a practice by which an ordinary person can achieve that state. Furthermore, it is usually clergy or leaders of various religions who purvey those texts. If they are womenless men, they often end up degrading the feminine. And without the feminine, the masculine is also degraded.

In John's case, his relationship to his wife *is* the nondual realization that he'd been seeking in his Vedantic studies and practices. His relationship to his own embodiment of merging masculine and feminine *is* his nondual practice. John now does the Promise on a regular basis. It has become a part of his spiritual life.

It doesn't need to be that way for everyone, of course. Some people aren't interested in a spiritual life. For them, the practice can stand by itself, without a religious context. Intimacy with one's own breath and skin allows the life force in the heart to flow through the entire body. That's the essence of the Promise and what the Promise sets free in each of us, and it's available to everyone.

Love Comes

As we have been seeing, the qualities of male and female are interdependent and mutually expressive. Within a partnership, the true pleasure of the male is in the pleasure of the female, not solely in the one-sided satisfaction of his own desire. It is vitally important that each partner be receptive to the physical and emotional needs of the other, to strength receiving in the flow of feeling within and without.

The prior practices of body and breath give you this, I promise. In sexual union, the man's enjoyment increases as he gains the courage to acquire the sensitivity necessary to please woman. He is there for her as strength, but he also becomes a soft and receptive vehicle for her own movement. The deeper her release, the deeper his will be too. The female orgasm provides the depth for both bodies to open up to each other and connect viscerally. There is a fullness of life that moves within and throughout both the man and the woman. On an emotional level, the man surrenders to the woman and offers his love to her. She receives him and surrounds him with her love. He then has more love to give her, and she has more love for him. In this mutual surrender, the strength of both partners is gathered and permitted to flourish.

Consider Carol's experience of how surrendering to the feminine paradoxically increases the feeling of strength. She is married to a chiropractor and lives in Hong Kong.

I asked my husband, John, what intimacy felt like. John said, "I feel you everywhere, surrounding me, embracing me. I feel your breath, your strength."

"How does my strength affect you?" I asked.

John replied, "I feel powerful."

Our lovemaking is tender, sweet, and intuitive. At this point, my husband did not know how the Promise works. I would explain to him later.

Intimate lovesex (this is a new word, by the way) is not about rushing at each other, racing to have the fastest tension-release orgasm. That's okay, too, but there is so much more. Each moment is so pleasurable that you relax into the feeling, which is full and sufficient. Should orgasm arise, then it will not be depleting. Instead it is an energetic, pulsating thrill for the whole body, and will move through both partners. Men often sound envious that women can have multiple orgasms and keep coming back for more, but a man can also share the same bodily thrill as a woman without ejaculating.

In the Promise Practice, a woman learns to relax without needing urgent tension release. She then can enjoy as many whole body orgasms as occur naturally. Her partner will enjoy all of them. They are as much his as hers, because they are shared, and their mutual participation increases the energy of both. He learns to be responsive to her movements. He receives her energy and movement as she receives his. The receptivity of daily moving and breathing allows this special receptivity. It becomes an energetic play between the feminine and masculine qualities of each partner—between each other and within each. You respond to the masculine and feminine in your partner, as well as within yourself, creating an endless, spiraling exchange. Women can surrender in the traditional sense of receiving male energy or play an active role with a receptive male; and the same range of options is available to men. It is as true for same-sex intimacy as opposite-sex intimacy. You become more interested in whole body absorption with each other and with pleasuring your partner instead of fulfilling your own pleasure. The base of the body, just as in the Promise exercises, cooperates with the whole body, or heart, rather than having an urgent life of its own. Likewise, your head gives way to the heart instead of having an imaginary identity and contrived social images of its own. The nurturing flow of feeling circulates through both hearts like shimmering flowers opening to each other.

A Friend's Birthday Card to His Wife

Dear Rose,
Root standing in your ground, I feel your earth, a certain scent, the ground where your roots spring forth intertwined with mine. Above you flowers are blooming, and I collect their nectars and subtle energies into my spine. My own root sap springs forth into the tips of my petals and graces the ground where you stand with the power you give me. I feel this even now on the

opposite side of the earth. Thank you, my nearest
and dearest, for delicious kissing like you mean it.
   All my love,
   Peter

In mythologies of many traditions, woman is Goddess, who is both a nurturing mother and the active force embodying the power of birth, life, and death. She is the power of reality itself. And nothing makes a woman feel her Goddess more than whole body orgasm, revealing her power to herself and her partner. The job of the male "God" is to serve the feminine and provide all her needs. This makes him feel his God. Obedience to God is in receptivity of the feminine, not control of the feminine. The overall principle is that the pleasure of the male is not in fulfilling his own desire, it is in the pleasure of the feminine. Electric impulses travel up the spine to the brain, which then triggers orgasm. Sometimes we think of sex as something purely physical, but on a neurological level, the intelligence of our bodies is registering the millions of nerves that are being stimulated and that allow us to experience bliss—a perfect example of how the symphony of cells in our body works in our best interests! The nerve ends seem to uncurl to allow the essence of our hearts to spring forth to each other, flooding body and mind with a healing spirit.

Men tend to think of orgasm as a single event, because that's how most men experience it. Individual orgasms may vary in intensity, depending mainly on how stimulated or tired you are, or even the time of day, but that's about it. Yet we have known for some time now that women experience a kind of progression, from clitoral orgasm, to vaginal orgasm, to whole body orgasm. For most women, it's helpful, if not essential, to begin with clitoral stimulation and perhaps clitoral orgasm, with or without male penetration, and build up sensation through the vagina and finally the whole body. Some sexologists and other teachers dismiss the clitoral orgasm as being lesser, and promote deeper, whole body orgasm as a goal. But there is no goal, and many women report powerful climaxes just from initial clitoral stimulation. There is also a particularly helpful place for some women to be stimulated just inside the upper vaginal wall, sometimes called the G-spot. All these areas and levels of stimulation overlap to some extent. There is no right way, and the key to intimacy from a male perspective is to be attentive to how your partner responds at each level—and to be bold to be there. Bold enough to please.

On the subject of female sexual satisfaction, Dr. Kim Wallen, PhD, a professor of behavioral neuroendocrinology at Emory University, has made a lifelong study of sexual response. He was once asked to name the most important thing he had learned in all his research. "Pay more attention to females," he replied. "My first great insight was that females are actually telling males a lot that males aren't paying attention to." The implications are huge for our personal and public lives, as we participate more in the natural state and the natural collaboration between the sexes. The focus on caring for the needs of the feminine, mother, Mother Earth, and all her offspring brings peace to everyOne. I am not suggesting that we return to a primitive state. We are an extraordinary species. Our crown and frontal line are designed for feeling and receiving, supported entirely by the masterful strength of our base and spine. You will feel this impeccable male-female design of the living organism in the Promise Practice. We *are* in the natural state of life, and to live well and even to survive, we need life's gender solidarity and teamwork with these extraordinary bodies!

Indeed, the whole body is an erogenous zone, and most women *and* men respond powerfully to being touched or caressed in places other than the genital region. It's all about opening bodies to each other, to receive each other's strengths, gifts, and subtle energies. That is what the Promise Practice prepares you to do, because it's all about your whole body being able to feel all that can be felt, opening yourself to life and love through breath and movement. It is whole body absorption one to another in the flow of life. This is the meaning of "love thy neighbor as thyself" in its most vital essence, revealing the great gift that life offers. As I've said, becoming intimate with yourself allows you to be intimate with another in new and extraordinary ways. Just as you learn to love your own breath and allow it to merge with your movement during the practice, you can do the same with your partner during physical intimacy.

Having gone beyond the urgent need for tension release, a man allows his and her natural chemistries and energies to flow and merge. He allows her sincere feminine force to be his. It is an adventure and a gentle progression that can continue for a lifetime. Humor and mutual agreement are the obvious moods of the adventure, with great respect for the unique qualities and needs of each person. The best advice might be, "Don't take anything seriously, except caring for each other."

I suspect that the reason so many women report feeling unsatisfied—despite all the how-to sex videos on the market—is that many men are either too self-absorbed or simply lack the knowledge of how to be receptive to a woman's pleasure. And society is so busy doing everything else as a substitute for what we really need: intimate connection! Part of the reason for that goes back to our social prejudice against sexuality as an obstacle to spiritual achievement, or the exaggerated stereotypes of what constitutes good sex. Until we learn to engage our sexual desire as intimate connection, though, we'll never realize that it is in itself a form of spiritual practice—perhaps the highest form we have. When both partners acknowledge and honor their sexual needs, their emotional, energetic, and psychological natures intensify in spirited connection, and what could be more spiritual than that?

Amazing intimate sex requires more than martinis and magic, then; it is a result of the Promise Practice of love and mutuality. When you have intimate lovesex, you cherish it for its ability to connect yourself to another body, to melt into and become absorbed in another whole being. The bodies know what to do. It is like writing in a new language without words. Pleasure springs from the flow of desire and the circulation of energy feeling between mutual lovers, not in the fulfillment or ending of desire. In the current social context, this idea may sound unusual, but men can bypass orgasm while still full of desire and see what happens. Do this and experiment with the frequency of ejaculation—less often for an older man than a younger man. Love and embrace each other as the whole body, and allow the base to be in coopera- tion with the heart and head rather than having an urgent independence of its own. Embracing from the heart and head, allowing attention to rest in the crown above, tends to move the regenerative force of life through the whole body, base to crown, from the heart, without depleting you or spilling energy from the body base. This allows you to relax as the whole body and prolong the pleasure for your partner. As she goes deeper, you go deeper in whole body love. The energy release through both after the feminine orgasm is particularly potent and worth the time spent in strong and gentle receptivity. It is worth gold and can be a unique experience, because instead of a tension-release orgasm, energy and desire remain a regenerative force even when you are apart. As time goes on, that force of regeneration is felt to be active in you and in the relationship itself, without there necessarily being a physical exchange. Inevitably, intimate occasions may not occur as often, and may or may not be an imperative for couples. Regardless of frequency, the relationship itself is a source of refreshment and nurturing.

Please discuss this openly with your partner, and use the Promise to explore your intimate potential. This is a special male responsibility, because strength does the receiving here, just as it does in the Promise Practice. The union of the male-female polarity enacted as the breath cycle within translates immediately into this capability of receiving each other. The male collects and allows for the strength of the other to flow out in an endless exchange of feeling. We give and receive. We are there for each other as strength in synchronistic and equal receptivity. We must correct the social imbalance that has been imposed on the perfect balance of our biology that is sex, the utter union of male and female. This union, love itself, has been taken from us through religious idealism, and people make less of their lives by trying to feel it in inappropriate ways, or they just give up. There must be a practical way. The Promise will give all this to you and your partner. You cannot attain it merely on an intellectual level as a good idea without practice, yet it comes as a natural gift of your easy daily promise.

If you do not have a partner, bring yourself to the point just before orgasm and allow yourself to relax into the feeling. Stay there for a while. Practice this regularly, as you would if you were making love in a relationship. It is making love to life itself. Explore the power, beauty, and bliss of your own body. Being familiar with your energy and sexuality prior to a relationship will help you develop a sex-positive attitude. Self-pleasuring can be used positively to liberate yourself from negative social restrictions and to become entirely affirmative in your sexual response. Just go ahead. You are going to feel relaxed, open, self-accepting. It is a kindness to yourself. It can also be helpful for couples in developing sensitivity toward each other. Only through the positive embrace of sex, with or without a partner, can we remove the pain of past suppression. If celibacy arises, which it inevitably does for everyone, it should be natural, without motive.

Although a vital part of intimacy is spending relaxed time together, other than the daily chores of life or lovesex on occasion, you also need to spend time alone, when you can feel the integrity and completeness of your life as an individual. Too much constant company or overfamiliarity can diminish the energy between the polar opposites. Time apart allows you to build up your individual electric charge, so that when you do get together, the power of opposite attraction will be stronger. You may spend that time with other friends, on personal projects, at work, and even days away from home, all of which are vital in maintaining the integrity of an independent life. The best relationships are built on the association of autonomous individuals who choose freely to be with each other.

There is a codependence in nature, the power of life that creates new life. To acknowledge this does not need to create social codependence: when two people cannot exist without constant reference to each other, and the dramatization of each other's imagined limitations siphons energy away from the relationship and its enormous potential. The intimacy of the Promise Practice with one's own body, breath, and life gives this autonomy and allows a person to choose and come to the partnership with energy and full participation.

If there are problems between you and your partner, start to heal them now. Reach. Touch. Practice intimacy daily. By allowing your energy to move toward
your partner, you will soften the restriction in your own
heart, body, and mind, clearing the pathways within and
without. Make a physical link, and the energy will move
between you as love. But don't make orgasm a goal! In
sincere friendship and feeling, things happen. You are
dealing with the entire human history of sexual restrictions and misconceptions that have been handed down
to you. So take your time. Don't search. Don't rush. Some
women may never orgasm like others. That is their consti-
tutional makeup, and there is no necessity for it. Men may
lose their erectile capability in the natural cycles of life.
It does not matter, and you should use pharmaceuticals
and other interventions cautiously. The cardiovascular
benefits of the Promise Practice will maximize your potential. But all can deeply relax and imbibe the intrinsic
body intimacy and resolve in the feeling of life. The Holy
Grail is in your own strong spine, in the receptive front
of your body and heart. That's where your life becomes
relationship and mutuality; and sex, the flow of Nurturing Source.

The practice is a daily reminder that you exist as authentic life, with love and the function of the universe
within everyone. You will not develop healing sexual
union without the prior practice of sensitivity to your
own body and breath. Otherwise all of this remains un-
fulfilled and disappointing, like any other ideal without a
practical means to attain it. We see disaster in countless

people's lives whose innate desires are stimulated with no means to practice intelligently. These woes will be with us until sex is known to be the spiritual practice it is, one in which we can engage intentionally. The good news is that the Promise Practice will give you what you need. Make it your priority.

CHAPTER 9

The Promise of Partnership
and the Promise in Partnership

Sex becomes sublime in the garden! Just wait and see!
Your base is united with your crown, your inner with
your outer, and you are making love with your world
in the mutual embrace of passion and respect.

WE ALL NEED TO MOVE BEYOND THE FAIRY TALES OF contrived love and the social pressure to find a partner and develop a sincere, lasting relationship. Your Seven-Minute Wonder is a short and achievable practice that will allow you to develop the necessary sensitivity to receive another in an intimate relationship, and the practical means to develop and sustain it on every level. It is a catalyst for entering into relationship, helping you become strong for others and receptive to others. You can cut a pathway through society's dysfunction and find somebody who is compatible with you. By choosing to engage in this process, you learn to value your partner as much as you value yourself. Your practice is the gift of touch and connection. It is desire and attachment—the natural giving and receiving of life's energetic flow. It is compassion in action: breath, movement, and making love.

Relationships require investment and commitment, and the desire and intention to connect with another is a beautiful and necessary part of life. To ensure that your intimate relationship is supportive and nurturing for both parties, you must be ready to acknowledge sex and intimacy as essential parts of the human experience. That requires releasing any ideas that limit your ability to feel and relate. You have it completely within your power to create a nurturing and supportive reality that is inclusive of your intimate partner—you simply have to stop looking and start living.

Fiona's Story: Space to Develop Intimacy

Following the Promise has, in a most real and tangible way, revealed and enhanced a deep fullness and intimacy between my partner and I. These simple yet profound teachings, so easy and enjoyable, have opened up an untapped depth of relationship I had always longed for but had previously found elusive. From my heart, these words are for everybody who, like me, desires to be connected to his or her true and natural state. As each soft breath is received and released, I feel like I am drinking from an eternal well—the very source of life—that I see to be in us, as us, and all around us. This connection to breath, this breath that is life, I feel deeply in my body, in the heart of my heart, expanding and encompassing an exquisite, innate joy of intimate love and connection with another. It is so effortless and natural, breathing together, moving together, participating in the dance of life together. Separateness and boundaries dissolve as he surrenders himself to me, and I receive him wholly. I feel his love move through me, as me. This is the essence of sex as love, of knowing another as yourself. Strength and softness received from simply inhaling and exhaling, being with body, being with breath. And sharing this with another is to be with life itself—life enhancing, life enriching, a promise of the extraordinary in the ordinary life we share.

Our spiritual growth depends on our resolving this real need for connection and intimacy. We are alive, and there is no need to prove ourselves otherwise. Once our attention is focused on what we truly desire, it will move us naturally in the direction of our choice. To ensure that this comes about, make the promise to practice both to yourself *and* your intimate partner. When you join in union with another, a third, powerful entity is created that is fully expressive of the vitalizing energy that is flowing through us and around us. Your practice is your active participation in this source, allowing you to recognize and embrace your place within the context of the whole, and freeing you of any restrictions that may have previously prevented intimacy from arising. Admitting to your partner that you are more powerful with her than without her, in the context of mutual expression and reciprocation, opens the channels for a deep river of feeling to be developed, as well as a divine reverence and gratitude for what each person contributes to the relationship.

Most of us limit ourselves from reaching this level of understanding with each other, and instead construct deep, protective layers to shelter ourselves from possible rejection and emotional hardship. Very few of us are brave enough to allow ourselves to be completely vulnerable in relationships, choosing instead to remain contracted and in a position where we believe we are in control. If you manage to shift your focus slightly, your eyes can open to the power that vulnerability allows. From here, you are "unlocked" enough to see clearly your own restrictions and limitations. By acknowledging and moving beyond them, you move closer to the truth and, consequently, closer to the power of life. When you are at your most vulnerable, you become your most "real," and you open up to an authentic experience of life and love. You become receptive enough to absorb the energy and love offered to you by another, while also being free of any barriers that may have previously prevented you from sharing your love openly. This is honesty in its purest form. From there you can enjoy the peace and power that emanate from within you and concurrently enjoy life's movement toward your partner.

In your Promise Practice, it will become clear to you that the physical experience of body and breath, strong base and spine with soft crown and front, is intrinsically linked to all other forms of experience, including and especially intimate relationships. We release what is old on exhalation to receive what is new on inhalation. The exhalation assists in the immune function of the system. It strengthens and supports all the lower organs responsible for life's elimination function, massaging and heating the body base. This helps life to reject what's not needed for your health, strengthening the male aspect of your life. The inhalation fulfills the feminine aspect of life, giving us the nurturing that we need.

Similarly, our relationships—which are the dynamic exchange of energy between two people—require this ongoing process to remain healthy. We need strength and receptivity in equal measure, which come through in the balancing of male and female within us, and within the relationship. Traditional roles that see men as only "strength" and women as only "receptivity" have been shown not to work. It is now time to get things back into balance.

Many women report that after doing the Promise, they can feel their strength as women growing and expressing itself for the first time. One friend said the only other time in her life that she'd felt such permission was in childbirth, when the men in her life had to organize themselves around her needs and receive her great power. Her strength as the nurturing giver of life was served by her partner's interest in receiving her strength. Her life-giving and nurturing power was freed up and allowed to come forth in full expression. At all times, women should be able to experience their full life-giving potential as the moving breath within them. The mother-father love that arises from the male-female polarity is the natural state of life and is as simple as the inhalation and the exhalation. This is the practice of love, and it allows you to enjoy love throughout your whole life.

Crescence:
A Midwife's Story, Sex and Spirit

After I gave birth for the first time, I didn't have words for what I had experienced, but I knew for certain that I'd had the strength to let the power of life move through me, and I knew that in its wildness, love was alive. I'd had some doubt, you see. What followed was a depth of connection between me and my daughter that took me completely by surprise. I had expected to meet a stranger, and yet this person with a face as round as the moon was someone I knew. Our knowledge of each other has spanned twenty years now, and it is beautiful.

I have now been given words for this beauty, and a practical way to nurture it and be that power for another. I am Source. I am Mother. I am simultaneously and completely sexual and spiritual. My power is love, and it flows in relationship, and this is my usefulness as a Yoga teacher and a doula. I was at a birth a few days ago with a couple who were in a dreadful place. Through the course of labor, the woman made friends with her body, and as she did, she was able to make friends with her husband too. As she gained the courage to know herself as a sexual being, she welcomed him in his wholeness. They opened to each other. This is how their child was conceived, and it was essential for its birth. We are all born out of love. It is indeed our natural state, something so simple that it continues to leave me speechless.

The experience of love that starts with the male-female union and manifests as new life should be our blueprint for relationships. We have been blessed with an extraordinary physical body that is capable of an enormous depth of feeling, and it can assume its place naturally in complete integration with all natural forces. Our breath and the inherent power of male and female intimacy are powerful realities that should be felt and enjoyed. By engaging in your practice, you become both strong and receptive—strength receiving—which allows for intimacy with your body, breath, and partner. As a result, the exchange of sexual energy will take its most natural place in its most natural form. The Promise of moving and breathing allows for this.

The Promise Without a Partner

In no way am I making a case for any necessity of relationship or sex. It's just that this is how nature operates, and so most of us are likely to be taking part in this regenerative exchange of energy between opposites—the source and power of life. If sex diminishes naturally, as it does in time, so be it. If we find ourselves in a state of motiveless celibacy, well and good. To prescribe sex or celibacy as strategies to one day gain entry to some imagined, amazing place, heaven or enlightenment, forget it! While the energy of sex is naturally moving in us, it is best to find a way that is right for us to participate. As I said earlier, nature has only one interest: the survival and evolution of the species. Let that speak for itself.

If you find yourself without a partner, for whatever reason, don't worry. During the course of life, most of us are without a relationship or partner at some point or another. Rather than viewing it as a negative event, consider it a special advantage or blessing. This is, in fact, an opportunity to recover; to embrace other aspects of life and relationships in a way that is sometimes not possible when partnered. You have the chance to devote time and energy to many people and pursuits. The link between you and Nurturing Source Reality is not weakened through this experience. Love is enacted between you and the universe. Here is a wonderful time to enjoy your autonomy, as well as all forms of intimacy.

It is also important to think about the ways in which you end relationships that no longer have the necessary love energy required for them to continue. Often separation is a sad experience, and in the process of reestablishing individuality, couples add complications by saying and doing things that make the pain even worse. Our language and behavior may be mostly reactive, and may come from a place of sincere sorrow, but our expression of it through anger and hostility distorts this. Again, this scenario is a result of social dysfunction, and we have not been given adequate language and methods to disengage respectfully from an intimate partnership in a way that honors the magical connection that once existed. Just because the need to share life in the context of a partnership has ended, it doesn't mean that you should devalue what the two of you shared. We do have the ability to end intimate relationships with dignity, and this is something that the

Promise Practice helps you to do. In the difficulties of separating from someone, it is hard not to take it personally and view it as a failure, but please understand that society is dysfunctional in the area of male-female polarity. Many of us have not had sufficient models of adult intimacy to understand true intimacy. When all the loving that can be done has done its healing work, yet obstructive patterns persist stubbornly between two people, it is sometimes necessary to recognize this and to move on, and do your loving elsewhere. I'm not suggesting that you do that casually, just as you didn't come together casually. But honor it as a sacred parting, in gratitude and respect for the relationship and all that has been achieved and all that you've shared. From there take it in your stride, and do your loving in the present, not in the sentimental past.

During your time without a partner, the role of platonic love may come to hold more importance. Love relationships that are not sexual are quite powerful, whether between the same or opposite sex. Take this window of opportunity to view more autonomously the sexual negativity that you may have absorbed unconsciously from familial or cultural sources. You may have noticed that when you go camping in the wilderness, or live through an extended power outage because of a storm, you have a chance to reevaluate your relationship to the electric and digital worlds, both to appreciate the benefits and understand the implications of dependency. That doesn't mean that you suddenly decide that you want to spend the rest of your life in a cabin in the woods with no Internet, TV, or refrigerator, but you do see things a little differently.

Likewise, the absence of a primary romantic relationship can provide an opportunity to develop these other relationships and discover how deep and special they can be. And if you are able to share the Promise Practice among friends, you may be able to allow it to become the context in which you and your friends can consider the sincere need for relationship.

Personal autonomy and partnership go hand in hand. Understanding the power and potential of relatedness is the starting point. Enter into relationships in the light of mutual appreciation and commitment to love as the whole body. It will make all the difference in terms of your intimate relationship. When we're not seeking sex or saddling it with philosophy and dogma, then we can experience a world of abundance—like those male and abundant female papaya trees spilling over each other. So without seeking, reach over and be with somebody who is right for you. Do *all* you can do to cut through the dysfunction of society.

My teacher would say this: if you want two things, then you won't get either. But if you know what you want, no power in this world can stop you. So choose what you want, and move forward in that direction with continuity. Life will provide you with all the nurturing you need.

Being Permissive About Sexual Choices, and the Garden of Eden

I was a small boy—about eight years old, as I remember. I lived in a romantic world of childhood mysteries, as my eyes and ears opened to a beautiful life of perfume and color, mother-father love, and the early reveries of being born in a New Zealand Garden of Eden. Two beautiful sisters about my own age lived next door, and they too were enjoying the delights of trees and flowers and all natural things. My bedroom window overlooked their driveway. Now, these two little girls used to have lots of fun running from their front door up the drive, past the hedge, and to the roadside gate. They would giggle and almost show themselves in the street and run back laughing. And they did this naked! A risqué game of show and run, a sensual rollick that one small boy witnessed delightfully without being noticed.

Innocently, I told my schoolboy friends the next day what I had seen. When asked what they were like, I replied, "As juicy as a peach," the closest description in my experience. Somehow this story got to my teacher and on to the headmaster. They started shouting, scolding me for what I had said. Everyone was in a state of panic and shock. My mom and dad were even called in to deal with this very bad boy. I knew then that it was a world gone wrong.

The innocence of the girls and the young boy was suddenly replaced by society's negativity toward sex. Only many years later was I able to see the total picture of life denial and man's pervasive destruction of the natural state. The fruit in the garden is for tasting! The universe has given us the apples and the "peaches" for our nurturing sustenance. The Adam and Eve story needs to be retold from a different point of view. From man's fear comes the attempt to own, know, and control our natural resource. This fear destroys our natural state of enjoying our sexuality, and this is the original sin; this is what is meant by "don't taste the fruit." Rather than control resources, we can receive resources. Rather than controlling the feminine, we receive the feminine and let her thrive. Inhale! Inspire! Receive! That we all return to the garden, indeed, in the context of man-woman mutuality is possible because it is the natural state.

Years later, when I realized this truth, I began to engage in the process of renewing intimacy in every way, until even sex would become utterly positive, the expression of love and life. When the male strength becomes receptive to the feminine, both man and woman become stronger, more durable, intelligent, and resourceful.

In our world, many kinds of exaggeration and dysfunction have arisen around sex precisely because sex is life's most powerful inborn force. It is as powerful as breath. Stop breathing and see what happens. You'll feel like you will explode. Sex must have its way and function. We are all meeting this natural force as best we can. There is no rule book, no "shoulds" or "should nots," and everyone's sexual journey deserves our tolerance and compassion. From celibacy to sex addiction, from abstinence to pornography, from frigidity to promiscuity, from casual hookup to crippling codependence, everyone is responding to the given reality of sex within society's confused interpretation of it. Even criminal outbursts must be seen in the context of the social disease, and we must nurse and educate the abused and the abuser back to positive life.

Through all of this, one thing is true: sex is completely natural, and we can carve out a path of intimacy and sexual wisdom for ourselves *because* it is natural. Every-One can enjoy intimacy with life by connecting with his or her own body and breath. Right now, you can experience intimacy with the male and female polarity that is in you. If sex does not occur, it does not matter. You still have intimacy.

Merge the inhalation with the exhalation; it's as simple as that. It can feel like your right side is fucking your left side. Really! Above to below, the utter eros-love connection. You will feel the complete mutuality of all the opposites of your life in a continual union and energizing relationship. That's a Promise.

Amy Bankoff's Story: Partnership Within Partnership

Since doing my Promise Practice, I've found ease in balancing life's rhythms. I've gained self-confidence, contentment, and the ability to accept fully whatever or whoever is in front of me. Most important, my Promise Practice has improved my relationship with my husband, which naturally has had a positive impact on my children.

In my practice, I've awakened to the innate, pleasurable connection with my breath and body, my inhalation and exhalation serving each other and the power they possess together.

This sensitivity, which we're all born with, eluded me for so long because I kept trying to find it. My feelings of self-doubt and worthlessness stemmed from my constant searching, striving to reach some goal of "perfection" or follow a method that others had convinced me I needed in order to be "better." Only when I stopped listening to others and simply breathed my body to move, did I awaken to the amazement within, to what has always been the essence of life.

From a young age, I felt the need to be someone beyond who I was. There was always a lacking, a desire to be skinnier, smarter, richer, more popular. I didn't allow myself to be a truly strong, confident woman until, paradoxically, I softened to life's natural ways. Since doing my practice, the need to struggle, to constantly be going somewhere and achieving something, has finally disappeared. I can feel my feminine side in ways I never have before. By inhaling deeply the full, embracing power of each breath, I've opened up to the gentleness with myself that I needed and craved for so long. And I've finally learned to truly accept whoever I am in each moment.

My relationships have also changed as a result of my peace becoming stronger. There was a time after I had my two children when having sex simply wasn't important for me. My husband, however, felt quite differently and our sex life—or lack thereof—brought anguish into our relationship. He wanted it, I didn't want to give it, and I thought it was simply a matter of my having no libido.

When Mark explained how the sexual relationship between a man and woman is the most important, most powerful aspect of a couple's relationship, my husband's frustration became very logical to me. Mark taught me that my sexual relationship with my husband is my most senior practice, the outer unity of the feminine and masculine in my own life—and I instinctively knew and felt this to be true, for it's how new life is created.

I began to engage with my husband, even when I didn't really feel "in the mood," and soon my desire for him was back. In a way, our sex life was like stretching muscles that hadn't been used in a very long time—quite difficult at first, with some resistance to even trying. But after a short time, the passion and pleasure of moving were reignited.

My husband began doing his own practice, and now, when the two of us lie together, there is a spontaneous movement of our bodies that is arousing. Thus, our sexual life has become an extension of our Promise Practices. Intimate connection on every level has been the ultimate gift for us through this practice. We have it with each other now, as well as within ourselves. We express ourselves more clearly and listen more carefully. We've become more understanding, patient, and forgiving with each other, and this is the gift of the Promise Practice: the always-present gift of real intimacy with life.

Love Clears Its Own Path

Once you experience a loving relationship that is expressed with the whole body, you will begin to see all the loveless patterns that have been programmed into you by society. Then you may experience difficulties in your relationship. The Promise offers a tried-and-true means of handling these difficulties when they arise in any intimate relationship. That is, you continue your daily Seven-

Minute Wonder, and you and your partner continue your bodily loving as frequently as you both decide is right for you. Only bodily loving removes the negative life patterns that we have inherited from previous generations. You have a means to practice your loving: body, breath, and relationship, in that order. Once you discover that the exhalation loves the inhalation as strength that is receiving the male-female quality of life, you will immediately feel an uncommon pleasure in relationships. You will love your partner with an utter connectedness, like the body loves its own breath. Sex is no longer limited to the stress-release activity of the conventional orgasm. You become more interested in fulfilling your partner by receiving his or her strength and movement. You become sensitive to each other in a sublime way.

Francesca: A Young Italian Mother

Throughout our fifteen-year relationship, my husband and I have experienced connectedness on multiple levels: physical, emotional, intellectual, and spiritual. This has changed and evolved over the years. Since practicing the Promise, it's as if we choose each other every day, asking why we are together, what connects us to each other.

I practice and teach the Promise regularly. My practice helps me to find my source in my heart, and to trust the heart as the driving source of my actions, thoughts, and communication. Being connected to my heart facilitates communication with my husband; it helps remove barriers, speaking truthfully and openly. I try to practice every day, when I find the right time. Some days it can be between three and three thirty in the morning, after my one-year-old son has woken me up and I can't fall back to sleep. I do quite simple moving and breathing, according to the time of the day, the phase of my menstrual cycle, how I feel, and the kind of stimulation I want to achieve, whether it's more energizing or relaxing. At the end of my practice, a quiet, introspective state often occurs spontaneously. I find myself engaged with different "objects," such as my son's smiling eyes, the flow of water, or a landscape. I often connect with love as an object, exploring the feeling of love resonating in my body—from the root of the spine to the top of my head.

My husband likes practicing simple moving combined with breath on a daily basis. He has discovered his breath and its boundaries, and how his body movement responds to the breath. Being an intellectual type, his Promise practice has helped him embrace his body and the corporeal manifestation of his feelings and emotions. And so he embraces me in a new and wonderful way. So, too, our relationship has changed, becoming more sensual; somehow more real.

Lovesex is not about technique or special skill. What matters most is allowing the quality of strength to equal the quality of receptivity in your loving together. Start where you are. Don't try to be something you are not. Be intimate with what you have. When partners practice the Promise together, they agree to "show up" for each other in order for the relationship to work. Sometimes, of course, our emotional state makes us reluctant to show up. For this reason, the Promise Practice can be viewed as a discipline, like brushing your teeth or taking a shower—something that you do regardless of emotions. When you do this, you find that you can easily turn up and be present to others.

Teaching and Partnership

To be clear, we realize the nature of life, our Source, and ourselves by embracing our experience. By having a life, we know life. Then we may very well become established in a natural certainty that everything is arising in absolute oneness or love. When we establish intimacy in our life, the beautiful ideals of religious abstraction—such as, "There is only God," or "There is One Reality in which all things are arising," or "Who am I without my negative story?"—become apparent. These insights come to us naturally and with stability in a life that is intimate. They are just given. Indeed, we can reside as witness, where all things and thoughts are known to arise in consciousness only. But you cannot practice these methods willfully. They only arise naturally as powers or insights that are given to you in the context of your intimate life, when conditions are right.

So it is best to be relaxed about these methods. Taken out of context, they have been forced on the public too soon, without the more fundamental spiritual practice of intimate connection. So much teaching is offered from these idealistic, heady positions that are too cerebral or disembodied and not practical. Sincere people, who have had spontaneous, extraordinary experiences, give these teachings but do not understand, so they cannot teach the process of establishing an intimate life. Such people are indeed to be respected, and the teachings are useful. I call these methods late-stage refinement of a human intimate life. Any remnants of the mind's structures of imagined separation from reality may dissolve in these reflections. However, the principle way to know "the Knower"— awareness or consciousness itself—is an emphatic ancient statement: embrace your chosen object or direction with continuity. In union with the object, we know the object, yet in so doing, we also know "the One" who knows. And that is how we know ourselves, Reality, or Real God. How wonderful that humanity works so hard to make life work for everyOne.

We cannot bypass the life of intimacy and take heaven by storm, so to speak. Having spiritual ideals is futile without first establishing a human life of caring affection. This is the means of realization, and attempting to circumvent it for imagined high ideals causes only trouble.

The primary practice is the embrace of all ordinary conditions. Always, in all ways, the main spiritual method of humanity (in all faiths) has been the personal and mutual intimacy between real people. The Christian focus on Jesus as a personal friend, for example, can be powerful. The personal intimacy in the Eastern traditions between guru and student, Avatar and devotee, carries the same transformative power. Even when there is sophisticated, refined teaching, such as in Vedanta or Buddhism, the personal intimacy with the teacher is the primary transforming agent in these traditions. These profound relationships were not a replacement or substitute for all other relationships but were there to help students in all their connections to life. The teacher gave everyone the core intimacy with life via each body and breath as their key to transform all other relationships. In the ancient wisdom world of Judaism, there is no exclusive Avatar, yet all appearance is Reality or God, so it is another cultural expression of the same wonder of all.

And the teacher is a real person, not an imaginary person; a real friend, not a social or personal identity; a nurturing function of life, not a superior. Genuine teachers are not conventional authorities but communicate to you only with the authority of real friendship and real caring. They can be found anywhere and may be down the street! They do not teach for their own agendas but instead to empower you and help you find your way home—the way that is right for you. For example, their guidance will never exclude your need for intimacy, including sex. We become grateful to such people, as we are to anyone who is truly a friend. This is the real devotion and compassion valued by the traditions. Through those early years and all stages of exploring life, it is helpful to have a real friend with whom you can talk openly.

It is okay to try all your options or not. Indeed, this was acknowledged in the great traditions, and a time was given in early adulthood to explore life options and make informed choices over a long time as to what was right for you concerning lifestyle, sexuality, and relationship. It was called the *brahmacharya* stage of life, which means to be a student or scholar of life or Brahman (an ancient word for God), by way of the right relationship to life in every way, and especially sexuality. The word is often translated as "celibacy" rather than the exploration of right relationships. This incorrect interpretation—the ideal that we are supposed to go beyond desires instead of embracing desires as religious practice—has caused many problems. Celibacy has been promoted as some kind of superior state. It is not. Life is about making the right use of desire, not suppressing it. Celibacy was never a religious practice before mankind invented hierarchy and doctrine.

In the meantime, if you feel confusion about sex and relationship, that is absolutely fine and to be expected. It is natural to go through a period of uncertainty, especially in late youth and the early adult years. Many questions need answers, such as: Who is the most suitable person for me, or what are my sexual preferences? Even questions around gender issues may need answering—and these big questions take time. Some experimentation is natural, and mistakes can be made through trial and error. It is all as it should be as we learn about life. You don't have to be in a hurry because certainty comes later.

So there can be confusion as we dissolve and renew the limiting patterns that we inherited from society. There is nothing to do but keep on loving, keep on connecting: body, breath, and relationships, in that order. At around the age of twenty-eight, there is the possibility of standing in your own ground, blooming in your own garden as life, free of childhood patterning. You feel your place in this world. You know your directions, relationships, and desires, and know how to move on them in the way that is *right* for you. This is the meaning of the word *righteousness*. Not cleaving to a mere belief system that you have been persuaded to follow but truly enjoying the power that moves your breath and sex. If it takes more than twenty-eight years, who cares? Don't be in a hurry. Things are happening!

Rev. Robert Conover's Story

The Reverend Robert E. Conover and his wife approached me after a seminar to express gratitude for what they had received. With sincerity and scholarly exactitude, they explained how vital the information was for them in the total spectrum of their religious studies and practice. Reverend Conover believed that it would be very helpful for his church, the Presbytery of the Redwoods in Napa, California. He later wrote to me:

For thirty years, I have worked with wise spiritual directors who all rightly directed my search inward and encouraged me to "be present." Trying my best to follow their instruction, I kept looking around on the inside, hoping to probe deeper and deeper within and find the "answer." Yet only after beginning the Promise Practice did I realize what it means to be present and to genuinely deepen my connection to life and the gift of my faith. It might seem to the outside observer that the strength and flexibility demonstrated by Your Seven-Minute Wonder is purely a physical accomplishment.

But the real accomplishment is the connection found deep within oneself, invisible to the outside observer: it is the profound connection between the breath and the body. This connection is the heart of the Promise. The Hebrew, Greek, and Latin words for spirit—ruach, pneuma, and spiritus—are closely associated with breath. Indeed, we receive the gift of spirit with every breath we take. Spirituality is as ordinary as breathing. There is no distinction between our ordinary, every-day life and our spiritual life. We need to coin a new word with no hyphen—"spiritualityreality"—to express the very tradition of the Hebrew prophets and Jesus. Such a practice can be helpful to people of all religious traditions, as well as for those who do not identify themselves as religious. For Christians, it can offer insight into familiar sayings such as "the Word became flesh" or "the kingdom of God dwells within you."

The Promise can help increase our understanding of our own tradition and inform our practice. Take, for example, the familiar teaching of Jesus to "love your neighbor as yourself"—a teaching widely embraced even outside of Christianity. But the Promise can help us see something even more significant. This saying is set in the context of Jesus's being asked, "What is the greatest commandment?" His response was that the greatest commandment is to love God, and that the second is just like it: to love your neighbor as yourself. In other words, the first and second commandments are one. Loving the Divine, loving our neighbor, and loving ourselves are all one thing.

Such an understanding also sheds light on what it means to love yourself. It is not self-absorption or self-indulgence, but it has to do with a deep connection to spirit and each other. In this way, the practical help of the Promise provides deeper insight into the Christian tradition and the possibility of deepening our own life of prayer and action. Mark and his teachers said that intimacy with the ordinary life is the principal means of a spiritual or religious life. I do believe there is something very instructive for Christians in the Promise Practice. The first has to do with a deep sense of unity with God and all creation. Human beings are "created in the image of God"—so, there is an inherent Divine element in every human person. In the Christian celebration of the sacraments of baptism and Eucharist, we are dependent on the very fundamental elements of the earth for our life: water, grain, and fruit. God, Creation, and all of humanity are acknowledged together in unity through these two sacramental practices. And to be with our breath is to be with the One who breathes us. Secondly, the Promise asserts the importance of a regular, easy discipline. For example, the Rule of St. Benedict is a prayer tradition long practiced by many Christian contemplatives. A "rule," or "exercise," or "practice," serves to continually ground and transform our identity. Such practice is not a just a habit but a pleasurable, conscious, and intentional discipline that transforms human life. In this regard, Mark shines light on the need for a well-formulated daily practice to live the spiritual life—or better said, to live in spiritualityreality.

PART II

Your Seven-Minute
Wonder!

CHAPTER 10

Let's Dive In

It is not enlightenment we need, it is intimacy. It is not positive thinking or awareness we need, but intimacy. It is not God realization we need, but intimacy. Yet intimacy gives all of these.

WHEN WE EMBARK ON SOMETHING NEW, REGARDLESS of what it is, we often cling to a common myth that we must wait for the right time to begin. For example, to begin your seven minutes of moving and breathing each day, you may feel that you need to wait until you are "in the mood." This is a seemingly innocent assumption, but it serves no practical purpose.

Instead consider the possibility that the reverse is equally true. The initiation of an action can generate and cultivate a mood. Ask any hard-working artist: she knows that if she waits for inspiration, she may never create much of anything, but if she works at her craft every day, she gets in a creative groove. That groove will cure procrastination, cut through lethargy, shake up your unproductive habits—and before you know it, you'll be in a wonderful mood.

Sometimes it's best to dive into a new practice, so let's. And don't forget to visit page 265 to view the videos of the Promise Practice.

Moving and Breathing

"I wanted you to discover this yourself," my teacher said many years ago, "not just tell it to you like another abstract fact to learn."

As I now pass on this simple practice to you, I want you to experience it yourself, and by doing so, discover it, as I did. We have before us the challenge of words on a page; if I were there in the room with you, I could demonstrate what I'm about to teach you. But I assure you, Your Seven-Minute Wonder is not difficult. You'll catch on quickly, I promise.

Breathing with the Arms (Sitting)

1. Start by sitting comfortably in a chair.

2. Keep your legs hip-width apart and both feet flat on the floor.

3. Let everything settle: relax your shoulders and let your arms hang at your sides.

4. Now lift your arms out to the sides in a slow circle until your hands are touching above your head. Look up, see the hands. Now lower your arms to your sides again. And rest.

You will notice that as you were moving, you were breathing naturally, and your breathing was corresponding to the movement of your arms. For most people, the instinct as they raise their arms is to inhale, and as they lower their arms to exhale. This is logical. When your arms go up, your chest expands and fills with air. When your arms go down, your rib cage settles, and the air in your lungs is expelled.

What I'm saying is obvious, but we're not always aware of it. In the normal busyness of life, our breathing goes on without our having to think about it. But in this moment, while you are enjoying your practice, you're invited to notice your breath. And notice that your body's movements are connected to it.

This connection is a vital aspect of your intimacy with yourself. I've talked about this many times in this book, but now you're getting to experience it. So:

1. Lift your arms again, this time with awareness of the breath that you're receiving. Without it, you would not be alive, and so, the very action of receiving your breath is life generating and life sustaining. Pause when your hands meet above your head. Let the palms and fingertips join together softly. And allow the stillness of that newly received breath . . . to be.

2. Now lower your arms to your sides, and notice that your breath is leaving you. You will also notice that strength is required for this to happen. Notice where that strength is coming from. As you exhale, your stomach lifts, inward and upward. Can you feel that strength? It, too, is keeping you alive, by releasing your breath and making room for new breath.

3. So pause with your arms at your sides. Allow the stillness of the exhalation . . . to be. In the brief moment of that stillness, at the end of the exhalation, you are truly intimate with yourself. This is true as well at the end of your inhalation. In fact, the entire breathing cycle, in conjunction with your body's movement, is an action of intimacy. Enjoy it. It is a wonder.

Are you ready to go on? Let's do it.

Breathing with the Arms (Standing)

1. This time, please stand up. If you're unable to stand or if standing is uncomfortable, then remain seated. You can also lie down, if that's what your body requires.

2. Once again, you will raise your arms above your head. But before you do, allow your breath to go ahead of your movement. In other words, start to inhale, and *then* move. When your hands reach each

other above your head, keep inhaling. Let the inhalation last longer than the movement.

3. You have just created an envelope of breathing around your body movement. The breath began the movement and extended beyond it. You might say that your breath has embraced your movement. This embrace enhances the intimacy of your practice. The movement of your body, the gentle upsweep of your arms, is completely surrounded by breathing. Pause at the end of your inhale and let this be.

4. Now exhale slowly. Again, let the breath lead the way. A moment of breath, released by the strength that is lifting from below, and then lower your arms. Let the exhalation continue after your arms are at your sides. In this action, it is the exhale that has enveloped, or embraced, the movement. Pause and let it be.

What I just guided you through is enough to begin Your Seven-Minute Wonder. Yes, I can teach you other movements, and I will. But this complementary connection between breath and movement—receiving the breath when you inhale, and releasing the breath with strength when you exhale—is the starting point of all intimacy. By doing this practice every day as simply as you did it just now, this intimacy will strengthen and grow like a muscle that is exercised each day at the gym.

We'll come back to this practice, but for now, just let it settle inside you, whatever that might mean to you.

CHAPTER 11

Let's Take a Breather

*The ancients considered the breath to be the primary
critical function of the whole body. Not the heartbeat.
We can participate in and strengthen the breath. Enhancing the breath, therefore, enhances all other critical functions.*

IN THE LAST CHAPTER, YOU WERE INSTRUCTED TO IN-
hale while sweeping your arms above your head and to
exhale while lowering your arms. In each case, the breath
preceded the movement and extended beyond it. As we
continue, the same method of breathing will apply. It is a
basic principle of this practice. The breath starts and ends
the movement.

Now let's consider the way you're breathing while
doing this practice. There is a method I'm going to teach
you. It will help you to control your breath, and it will
deepen the experience of your practice.

Again, I'll make this as experiential for you as I can.

Breathing Method

1. In a relaxed standing or seated position, begin by taking a few normal breaths. Keep your mouth closed softly. Breathe in and out through the nose.

2. Instead of using the nostrils to inhale, as if sniffing a rose, see if you can regulate the flow of the breath at the back of your throat. You may find it helpful at first to open your mouth and whisper a soft *haaaaa* sound on both the inhalation and the exhalation.

3. After you have practiced this a few times, close your mouth again and see if you can produce a similar sound and sensation while keeping the nostrils passive. You will feel the air at the nostrils very lightly, but the airflow is regulated at the larynx. This may come easily to you, or it may feel slightly strained. Gradually it will evolve to a surprisingly instinctual and pleasurably soft experience.

One advantage of directing the breath this way is that the continuous sound provides you with a focus. Your mind will wander from time to time—that's normal, and you might as well accept it. By listening to the sound of your breath, you provide yourself with a clear and tangible "point of return" that you can use throughout the various stages of practice.

Let's try that again. Inhale and exhale through your nose, and control the regulation of the breath at the back of the throat. The motion of air vibrating in this space produces a distant, hollow sound—do you hear it? It has been likened to a baby snoring, or the sound of the ocean that you hear in a conch shell. It is peaceful and very relaxing.

This type of breathing also lets you control the length and quality of your breath. It's a useful tool, then, in your seven-minute practice. For example, you learned that the breath begins and ends the movement. Being able to control your breath makes this much easier, while helping you to stay focused at the same time.

You may also notice as you breathe this way that your abdominal strength is enhanced when you exhale. You're working with your diaphragm, which, as it lifts, works the lungs like a bellows, expelling the "used" air. Can you see how you're participating with your breath?

The breath is key to making a practice that is personal to you. It allows you to develop a profound appreciation of your connection with your own Natural State and your place within the vastness of the world and all that it encompasses. By participating consciously in the breath, you are linking directly to that which is breathing you, the magnificent force that beats your heart and moves you through the infinite cycles of life.

Jane's Story: Engaging the Breath

I can still remember the day when I first learned how to engage the breath. At the time, I had no idea how this breath could help alleviate the suffering I had been going through. "Come on," I thought at the time. "We all breathe!" I thought I needed much bigger help.

That day was the beginning of the most powerful practice I have been given. It permeates the rest of my life, and expands my heart and my relationships: the good, the bad, and the ugly. Peace from this specific practice soothes my head at four in the morning when I can't sleep and I'm afraid. Recently, strength from this practice allowed me to hold the hand of my lovely mom as she left this physical world.

Let's return to your own experience of breath within your practice. You've learned that breath always starts and ends the movement, and you've learned this method of breathing into the chest cavity controlled at the larynx.

Now, as you breathe, be aware of all four phases of the breath:

1. inhalation
2. pause at the top of the inhalation
3. exhalation
4. pause at the base of the exhalation

An important element of your practice is to engage and participate in all parts of the breath equally, with focused but relaxed attention. Try it now. Regulate the flow of your breath consciously. As you do so, start to lengthen the breath. Your throat breathing will help you here, enabling you to slow down the breath and extend it a little.

We'll add movement to this in a moment, but for now, just breathe. As the inhalation and exhalation lengthen and deepen, you can begin to direct the inhalation into the chest, and as you exhale, notice again the inward movement of your belly. The following will help to isolate these areas:

1. Place one hand on your stomach and the other on your chest. As you inhale, allow your chest to rise gently toward your chin, and your abdominals will extend naturally. Drop your head a little toward the heart, gently stretching your neck and spine. Allow your attention to rest at the heart.

2. Excellent. Now pause the breath at the top of the inhalation. That's it.

3. As you exhale, contract and draw in the abdominal muscles that lie between the pubic bone and the belly button. With your hand placed there, you will feel them. Let the chest settle naturally.

4. At the base of the exhalation, pause the breath again.

There. You've successfully lengthened all four phases of the breath.

You may be feeling relaxed and comfortable as a result, or it may take you a while. I remember that when I first tried this, I was impatient with myself. I attempted to forcibly manipulate the breath to the point where it felt strained. But as I continued to practice, I went easy on myself, and before long, this method of breathing began to feel natural.

Emmi's Story: Subtle Change

I'm at day twenty-seven of my seven-minute Promise Practice. There were mornings when I struggled getting on the mat, but that is when the "real work" comes, if I can even call that work. But work *in terms of gathering the energy to get up from bed. Things don't happen without effort, which is part of being fully engaged. Physically, I have never felt better. The change is subtle; the heavens did not open, with angels coming down. Instead I have it here, in me. What I feel now this twenty-seventh day is that I've stopped looking for answers—because I have forgotten the question.*

The breath is central to your practice. It is your primary tool and indicator during each and every moment. It "inspires" (the word means "to draw in air"), initiates, encases each movement made during the practice, and gives the movement fluidity and flow.

Attention to the breath also ensures that you do not push past your physical limits or create emotional stress. The quality of your breath is a gauge; when you lose the ability to breathe smoothly and with ease, you know that you have extended beyond the body's comfortable limits and need to adjust your practice accordingly.

And while the body is your most tangible energy field, your breath is the subtle link to all elements of life, both seen and unseen. The breath allows you to establish a relationship with every cell in your body. By harnessing its power, you become sensitive to the changes occurring within you on a daily basis, and this allows you to maximize your feelings of wellness.

The controlled use of the breath is also the tool that allows you to release ingrained patterns and habits and clear the mind. It forms a connection between what you can control at a visceral level and those intangible elements to which you are inextricably linked.

Through careful observation of the breath, you can fine-tune your practice in a way that is conducive to your present life situation, ensuring that you move forward in a positive, intelligent manner.

The main thing is to enjoy the breath as your guide throughout the practice. Let the breath be your teacher. It is the key to creating a practice that is personal to you.

CHAPTER 12

Let's Get Moving Again

*The Promise Practice gives you intimacy with your
own life and the autonomy from which your intimate
relationships become authentic or truly chosen. It is
then not merely an attempt to fulfill imagined needs,
or childhood and adolescent responses to life.*

Forward Bend

You will now add a simple forward bend to the breathing
method that I've taught you. But *add* is not really the correct word. The body movement *is* the breath movement.
This may seem like an abstract concept to you now, but
as you practice, I think you'll discover the truth of it.
It's a key point when practicing breath and movement
together.

1. Please stand up.

2. Begin by inhaling and raising your arms above your
   head. You've done this before, but this time, gently
   arch your back and look up at your palms cupped

167

together. When doing any back arch, the curvature of your spine should be smooth from the base to the crown, with no acute angles. Be mindful of this. You will be able to feel a pinching or jamming sensation if you have gone too far.

3. Now, as you exhale, bend forward from the hips, leading with the chest, and draw a wide circle around your body with your arms. You may feel as if you're doing a swan dive. Keep your knee joints loose and let them bend as much as needed, maintaining your center of gravity through the soles of your feet.

4. You're now bent forward. Your fingers may touch the floor or rest somewhere upon your legs; be aware of what is comfortable for your body. Keep most of your weight on the front of each foot, with your toes active on the floor.

5. That's good. Now inhale as your arms and breath take you back up. Extend up into a comfortable back arch, with your hands above your head. Remember that breath starts and ends the movement!

6. Repeat steps 2 through 5 four times. Then, if you're feeling comfortable, stay in the forward bend for four more breaths. Maintain the same breath ratio that you established in the movement. Keep your neck flexible, letting your head relax.

7. After four breaths in this position, let your arms and your inhalation bring you back up again. Arch your back, look up at your hands, and this time, as you exhale, gently cup your hands together and lower them until they're over your heart. Lower your head slightly and enjoy a few resting breaths.

Shelley's Story

I had been practicing various forms of moving and breathing exercise for a number of years, with some dedication, before I found the Promise Practice. My body had always responded quite well to other methods, but after some personal issues, I started to hold a lot of stress within my body. Psychologically, I noticed that I was becoming quite "hard," and felt like my demeanor had become overly masculine as a way of protecting myself emotionally. This attitude seeped into my ability to move and breathe. Whereas I had previously been agile and flexible, my body was responding to the condition of my mind and had become quite rigid and stiff.

When I discovered this practice, it took some time before the idea of strength receiving really made sense to me, but when it did, the effect was utterly transformative. The importance of both male strength and female receptivity within the same person became apparent. This felt so powerful and healing, especially after having always felt that I was swinging dramatically between one quality and the other: either obsessively "strong" as a form of control, or overly "passive" as a way of avoiding conflict. This time I realized that I had been doggedly pursuing some kind of masculine strength to protect myself. The strength had been keeping me stuck in my body—and in the broader context of my life.

Recently, I went to a regular class I attend and used the principles of the Promise. Without any conscious effort at all, my body moved easily and comfortably again—so much so that I felt a very real union of male and female energies inside. The receptive inhale gave birth to the strength in exhale, and both are one and the same. It was a powerfully intimate experience that culminated in a feeling of bright, swirling energy moving up smoothly from the base of my body, through the heart, and to the crown of my head. I felt an overwhelming sense of love and expansion, which I now realize is the result of strength that is receptive, male and female, above and below. These polarities unite at the heart, and I could literally feel it as love within me and for all life around me. The physical experience of this has confirmed the power of the Promise Practice for me.

You may be getting a sense of what I mean when I say that the body movement *is* the breath movement. Balancing the strength and receptivity of the exhalation to the inhalation creates the internal union of the masculine and feminine energies within our own system. The microcosm of the self serves as the channel through which other union can then occur. When this begins to happen, the effect is noticeable within the body and in other forms of relationship. Where there was imbalance, harmony and intimacy can be restored because there is no longer any division. The merging of opposites, which starts within the body, is the key to intimate connection to life.

Let's move on to another movement, incorporating the same method of breathing. This one requires a little more effort, so, again, use your breath to gauge your body's capabilities.

Striding Forward Bend and Back Arch

1. While still standing, take a comfortable yet strong stride forward so that one foot is placed ahead of the other. Ensure that both feet are hip-width apart and that there is equal body weight distributed through both feet, with your toes active.

2. Inhale with your arms by sweeping them up into a mild back arch where you can see your hands, still allowing your shoulders to feel spacious and loose. Allow your arms to open the chest. Most of the arch should be felt in the upper back and the front of the upper chest.

3. Exhale while bending forward, tracing your hands around your body in a circle and allowing your knees to loosen as your fingers touch the floor on the other side of the front foot. Repeat this four times, remembering always that breath starts and ends the body movement.

4. After your fourth breath, inhale up into a back arch. If you feel comfortable, stay in the standing back arch, with your legs still astride, for two to four more

breaths. There should be no muscle strain or struggle. Be with your breath in its quality of strength (exhalation) that is receiving (inhalation), and notice the four parts of the breath:

1. inhalation
2. pause at the top of the inhalation
3. exhalation
4. pause at the base of the exhalation

5. Now switch sides and repeat with the other leg. Take a few resting breaths if you need to, and proceed when you are ready.

A Note About the Heart

As you practice, you may have noticed that during certain movements, the head naturally and easily lowers to the lifting chest, gently stretching the neck and the spine. As this happens, the mind bows to its source, the heart. On exhaling, the strength of the base cooperates with its source, the heart, in a comfortable surrender.

The heart is the source of all opposites, the culminating point of the body and mind. All opposites arise from and return to the heart. The heart is felt in the participation of its opposites. You don't need to come to any "realization" about this; it is just something that naturally arises. In the union of one set of opposites, all opposites are served.

The power of these practices is not commonly known

at this time. Yet rest assured that in the physical union and connection of opposites through body and breath, you are working with powerful energy. Let the breath be your teacher. Obey your teacher, and let your heart be your guide.

So far, you've learned four postures, each one incorporating breath and movement: (1) breathing with the arms while sitting, (2) breathing with the arms while standing, (3) forward bend, and (4) striding forward bend and back arch. Let's do one more before leaving this chapter.

Forward Bend with Twist

1. Standing with the legs parallel to each, move your feet wider than hip-width apart. There should be equal weight through the front of each foot. Keep the toes active, lightly gripping the floor. You'll use a wider stride as you get stronger in practice.

2. Inhale raising both arms to shoulder height, keeping all the joints loose. Lower your chin to your lifting chest, with your head lowered to the heart. Pause after inhalation.

3. Start the exhalation before the body movement. As you exhale, twist and take your left hand as low as possible outside the right foot. (It can be touching the leg or foot, or placed on the floor, depending on ability.) Loosen the right knee and turn to look at the right hand stretched out above the body. Gradually

lengthen the pause after exhalation as you proceed through the practice.

4. Inhale as you lift and return to standing with your arms outstretched.

5. Exhale, this time twisting the right hand to the outside of the left foot, turning your head to look at your outstretched left arm.

6. Repeat for two to six breaths. Those who feel comfortable may stay in the downward position, increasing the twist as you exhale and softening the twist on inhale. You should always stay in the natural elasticity of the body and the breath. Don't go beyond what your body can do; it will eventually find its own way there.

7. As a counterpose, now do a gentle forward bend, with the knees and neck relaxed. Remain here for two to four breaths, and then slowly uncurl back into standing. Take six to eight breaths in all, emphasizing the pause after exhalation.

Well done. In the next chapter, I will teach you five more postures, but before moving on, take a resting breath or two, or as many as you like. It's there, and always has been, for you to enjoy.

CHAPTER 13

Let's Go a Little Deeper

To be yourself is very easy; you don't have to do a thing. No effort is necessary, and you don't have to exercise your will. But try to be something other than what you are, and you have to do many unnecessary things and struggle a lot. To be yourself requires extraordinary intelligence. You are blessed with that intelligence; nobody need give it to you, and nobody can take it away from you.

YOU MAY BE THINKING AT THIS POINT THAT YOU'VE been given enough instruction to fill at least seven minutes of practice—and you're right. You have Your Seven-Minute Wonder. You know how to breathe, and you know how to move through a number of seated and standing poses, which you can repeat as many times as you like. You're good to go.

But I'm inviting you to stay, so that not only can you learn a few more movements and increase the versatility of your daily practice but also learn a little more about the practice itself.

Let's review what you've learned already, by your own experience of the practice so far.

The Five Easy Pieces

1. The body movement *is* the breath movement.
2. The breath starts and ends the movement.
3. The inhalation is receptivity from above and expansion of the rib cage, above to below, front and back. The abdominals settle outward secondarily.
4. The exhalation is strength from the base, the abdominals moving the diaphragm in and up. The chest settles secondarily.
5. There are always four parts to the breath: inhalation, retention, exhalation, retention.

In every posture that you choose to include in your daily practice, all five of these elements can be applied—whether you're standing, sitting, or down on the floor. As you progress, they will become natural to you, and you'll rarely have to think about them.

Yeshai: A London Business Consultant

The short daily practice works for me like magic. When I practice, my whole day looks different. It helps me to channel information, and my feelings are above and beyond. Physically,

I "move" much better—feeling lighter and looking better! Emotionally, I feel stronger. I send and receive love in greater and faster quantities. Spiritually, it helps me to open up my energy and communicate better with the environment. It is my intimacy with reality. This Promise is probably the best single action that you can take, with the best possible results!

Child Pose and Cat Arch

1. For the next movement, position yourself on your hands and knees. If you need to, place a mat or a blanket on the floor for comfort. Always take care of yourself. Forgo this movement if your knees feel uncomfortable.

2. Arrange yourself so that your knees are slightly apart, placed underneath the hips, and the hands are slightly in front of your shoulders. You are on all fours like a cat. Spread each finger and push down firmly through the index finger and thumb in order to take the pressure off your wrists. Now inhale.

3. With your exhalation, extend your hips smoothly back toward your feet, keeping your arms and hands outstretched. Feel your spine lengthen, and keep your abdomen tucked in slightly.

4. On the inhalation, come back onto all fours, simultaneously dipping your belly so that your collarbones and tailbone are the highest points. Keep your neck

long, but do not arch the head back to the point where you're straining.

5. On the exhalation, draw in your belly and move the hips back into the crouch position, extending your tailbone back. Practice these movements slowly, with total attention on the quality and comfort of your breath. If necessary, you can rest between each repetition to make certain that the quality of the following movement is equal to the last. Take four to six breaths, emphasizing the pause after exhalation.

6. Repeat this sequence three to six times, taking as much time as required. The forward folding of the body serves to tuck the belly in and up and push the breath out. It serves the exhalation. The unfolding of the body and the back arch serves the inhalation. Again, look after yourself. If you experience knee pain, skip this practice. "No pain, no gain" is faulty instruction!

Reach for the Sky

1. From the floor, bring yourself back to a kneeling position, with an upright but relaxed spine, and your arms resting at the sides of your body. Upon inhalation, raise your body onto your shins and sweep the arms up from the front of the body until they are raised above your head. Let the breath lead the movement as the arms reach skyward.

2. While exhaling and drawing in your stomach, fold forward from the hips and sweep your arms behind you. Place palm in palm to the small of your back or your arms to the floor beside your body. You will be crouched like a child, the universal playful, prayful position. Rest completely at the base of the movement, relaxing into the space between the breaths.

3. With the inhalation, sweep your arms out to your sides, and, using the strength of your inward breath, allow yourself to come back up onto your shins, as if standing tall on your knees. Note: If you find this movement too strong for your lower back, simply roll up through the spine until you assume a similar position. Pause here momentarily before gently lowering back down to a kneeling position on the exhalation, with your arms resting at your sides.

Legs to the Roof, Arms Overhead

1. Lie down on your back. Keeping your hips and pelvis on the floor, draw your knees in toward the body. Keeping your shoulders relaxed and connected to the floor beneath you, rest your hands lightly on the corresponding knees.

2. With the inhalation, float the knees up and away from your body, extending your legs and feet above you as your arms extend smoothly up and to the floor behind your head. Pause here.

3. Exhale as you draw the knees back in toward the chest, as the arms return and the hands rest on the knees once again. Repeat as many times as comfortable. When you have finished, you can rest for as long as necessary, either with your feet on the ground and your knees bent, or with your legs outstretched completely.

4. Take about four to eight breaths, resting between each one if needed. Never lose the connection to the breath, which starts and ends the movement!

The Bridge

1. Lie on your back, with your knees up and your feet on the floor hip-width apart.

2. On the inhalation, lift your pelvis off the floor as your arms come over your trunk to the floor behind your head.

3. Start the exhalation before you move, and lower your pelvis to the floor as your arms come down to the sides of the body.

4. Increase the pause after each inhalation.

5. Repeat three or four times.

6. Be sure that the breath starts and ends the movement.

Restorative

This is the most restorative, regenerative practice you can do, and can either follow the previous practices or stand alone as a practice for recovery and nurturing.

1. Lying with your back and shoulders on the floor, place your bent legs on a chair, with your knees and hips bent at 90-degree angles and the full weight of your legs feeling supported by the chair. There should be no weight through your hip joint.

2. On an inhalation, raise both arms up and over the head. Some people can reach the floor behind the head, while others may simply go where they can without strain. This should feel comfortable for you.

3. Pause after you inhale, and then start the exhalation as you bring both arms gently back down over your head to the sides of your body.

4. Pause and inhale while extending your arms again.

5. Continue this for six to eight breaths, then rest with your arms on the floor at shoulder height. You can increase the length of the pauses after inhalation and exhalation as you go. Experiment with this. The pauses should not compromise the length of the inhalation or the exhalation.

You might like to repeat this two or three times. To put the legs above the trunk is very helpful to the heart and the whole cardiovascular system. As I noted earlier, a doctor friend of mine told me that there is really only one illness—stress—which manifests as many illnesses. So de-stress every day, and you will optimize your health.

A Most Vital Conclusion: Rest

The most important part of your sequence is to complete your Promise Practice by resting your whole body. This should be done every time, no matter how long you have spent in the previous practices. Enjoy this experience as the ultimate nurturing for the whole self.

1. Lie comfortably on your back and let the body release and relax, supported entirely by the floor or ground beneath you. The more you surrender to the floor, the more you'll feel supported by the floor. The more you surrender to life, the more you'll feel supported by life. And you are completely supported by life!

2. Relax your legs, which should be spread hip-width apart, and allow your feet to fall gently to the sides.

3. Relax your arms a little way from your body, with the hands turned palm-side up approximately twelve inches from the sides of the body.

4. Relax each finger and each toe.

5. Rest each limb in the whole body.

6. Rest the whole body in its context of stillness.

7. Let your attention move through the whole body, surrendering each part as you do. Rest deeply as the whole body, whatever the whole body is altogether.

8. Think of everything that you don't need for wellness and visualize it leaving the body, flowing out of the ends of your arms and legs, like radio waves to infinity. The body naturally throws out what it doesn't need. In the Promise, you are participating in this function, releasing physical, emotional, and mental obstruction.

9. For a moment, let your attention rest in the crown or even above the crown. Rest the whole body in the flow of life.

10. Remain here for at least two or three minutes, or much more to your heart's content. This seemingly simple practice is powerful, and if you miss this final resting, it's a bit like entering data in your computer and forgetting to save it. This restorative practice preserves the benefits of all the practices done before it, so that they become enmeshed in the memory of

every cell in your body. So even if you've done only one or two of the practices described above, never skip this practice.

At this time, you could include any cultural practices that are near and dear to you, such as song and dance, poetry, prayer, *puja*, mantra, or any liturgy that you love.

That's it. You now have a number of breath and body movements from which to choose. You may want to select a few each day, and vary the selection, or, if you feel like doing more than seven minutes, you can do them all. This is your practice, and your own intimate experience.

To complement what you have learned here, there are various resources available to you to study these postures and movements in video form. You can follow the complete sequence on the iPromise iPhone app, Android, or YouTube.

Nianna Bray, Psychologist: Simplicity and Beauty

How do I kiss the earth? How do I connect with life? I experience the answer in my daily practice as a gentle reminder. It keeps me honest. There is simplicity and beauty in the mundane. The ordinary and the mystical reveal themselves to me with each conscious breath, in moments of clarity when I feel and know myself from the inside. My daily practice is my daily meeting of self. I show up, I breathe, I move, and I connect deeply to what is. Union is meant to be experienced, and life is meant for living. I don't know what life I would be living without the experience of this practice.

Your Commitment to Daily Practice

When you begin to do Your Seven-Minute Wonder, it may take a little while to get through the natural tendency of your mind to avoid discipline. Keep at it and be persistent, because with time it will become a regular and cherished part of your day. When in doubt, remember this simple rule: *It is only a three-breath discipline.* You will usually find that the first three breaths come a little reluctantly as you break through your resistance. The fourth breath, however, always comes sweetly and powerfully. Then it's simply a discipline of pleasure, but a discipline no less. One of my friends told me that after committing to regular practice, his whole perspective on the "discipline" of practice transformed. Before, he'd felt like he was always *doing* his practice, but after some weeks of regular moving and breathing, it felt like the practice was *doing him*! The body's innate knowledge took over to the point where it felt entirely natural to move and breathe in this way, free of effort or struggle.

There is another reason to promise yourself to do your practice. Our social conditioning contains an inherent reluctance to be intimate. Because of this, we avoid the direct experience of our lives; then we wonder why we feel that something is missing. The Promise is your direct practice of intimacy with yourself, with others, and with life.

Masha, Actor and Yoga Instructor: Sacred Space

For the past decade, I have been drawn to sweaty group exercise classes that teased me with the promise of looking good in my jeans. Then, after I learned the Promise, I began to love my own practice, and made a promise to do it every day. I no longer felt I needed big group classes to be motivated to practice, and I realized that I already look pretty good in my jeans. Instead I was excited to step onto my own mat and discover what happens when I'm just alone with my body and my breath.

By simply taking time for myself to move and breathe at my own rhythm, I create this sacred space each day, which allows my joy to rise unimpeded to greet the world. I'm nicer to the dry cleaner, the checkout girl, and the valet, and, somehow, they are nicer to me. As an actor, I usually have audition anxiety, but since making the Promise, I have begun to love acting without any anxiety about the results. Ironically, I've booked every audition I've had since. My relationship with my partner has also improved dramatically. I seem to have become more loving and patient with him simply because this practice allows me to be loving and patient with myself.

I ask you to have the courage to be intimate with your own life, breath, and body—it will serve you in every way. Seize this real, tangible opportunity, for you will not progress with good ideas alone. There has to be a practical means: something that you *do*. This practice *is* the practical means that will bring about direct experience and realization of your ideals; direct intimacy with life as Nurturing Source Reality. Commit to it and embrace it with open arms and heart, and you will see its transformative power.

And don't merely tell yourself, "I will try to do it." That never works, because the statement means you won't *actually* do it. When you say, "I will," or "I promise," then you do. You show up to your life. I have found that people love to be asked to make the Promise because the moment they do, they take a solid stand in their own life. I ask it of you—and perhaps you would ask it of others who need and are ready for the Promise.

CHAPTER 14

Your Seven-Minute Wonder Explained

It is not a matter of changing anything. It is not even a matter of finding centeredness or locating the heart. The heart is always already perfectly there. It is just a matter of participating simultaneously in the opposites.

BY DOING THESE PRACTICES, YOUR BODY RECEIVES complete nurturing. The sequence of forward bends, back arches, gentle twists, and inversions (legs above the trunk) has been carefully designed by the very best teachers to include everything that you need. The lived intimacy of breathing in and breathing out as you move brings about a physical union of opposites. The process allows you to participate viscerally in the exquisite union of *all* opposites, starting with the body but creating a powerful change in all aspects of life, which comes about through continued practice. Though seemingly simple, these practices bring about untold peace and power.

Depending on your time and energy, you may choose to practice only one or two of the sequences described. What is here is just a small taste from a seemingly endless menu of combinations and possibilities. Regardless of what movements you choose, your aim is always to facilitate the movement of the breath within your body. No matter how simple the movements are, the benefits are equally powerful. The complexity of the movement is irrelevant, and even the most basic movements performed correctly (with the inhalation and exhalation starting and finishing the movement) are as profound as those that are perceived to be more complicated.

Do not let yourself worry about where your physical practice is in relation to others. What one person may choose will be different from what another person may choose. Remember, your practice is the intimate connection to your own body and breath, and therefore it is designed solely and specifically for your own body and your own breath. Your Seven-Minute Wonder and the movements that you choose to incorporate within it involve only those that are suitable for you as an individual. What's important is that the movements you choose are done to optimize your practice as a joyful and pleasurable experience.

After your practice, you may feel like resting quietly in natural meditation or continuing to practice the breath in a comfortable, relaxed position. Do not force yourself to sit if the feeling does not arise of its own accord. Meditation is a clarity that arises naturally, and is not something that you can impose on yourself. We practice for the sheer joy of participating in the breath, which, in turn, draws us in and enlivens us to the nurturing force that is life. Anything else that comes as a result is like an added blessing, one that many practitioners of the Promise experience.

Christina's Story

Once I taught the Promise in a beautiful cathedral in Switzerland. It was such an ideal place to share with people. A few days later, a participant named Christina emailed me and shared her experience as a first-time Promise practitioner. It was the anniversary of her sister's death.

I like to say some words to you about what happened last Wednesday in the cathedral. My English is not very developed, but anyway, I was very touched to realize that we can get to be at one by breathing. I received that feeling of love that is actually universal love. Love existing in my heart. I am doing my seven minutes every day now, and like this, I can receive or feel this love. I never gave any attention on my breathing, and it's so wonderful to breathe the universe that is a miracle—to learn this way and learn more about life, about me. Two years ago, I had breast cancer, and three years ago, my beloved big sister died of cancer. Wednesday was her birthday, and I felt better, so blessed and honored after your class and able to continue in this wonderful life. I would like to give you my thanksgiving from all my heart. I love you, I love life, I love myself (and it's all the same time), and the Promise will help me to trust in the wonder of life. Hope to see you again. With a blooming flower of my heart, Christina

Two months later, Christina contributed to my blog:

I visited the Promise seminar on the 21st of October 2009 in the Cathedral of Saint Elizabeth in Basel. It was actually my first lesson. I could feel how important it is to breathe and how strong we can connect with God—or whatever we call the source of our life. I fell into a unity, which I could enjoy very much. I promised to do seven minutes every day. And it gave me a lot. I think the practice in a church is great. We could take out all the benches and make the churches (and ourselves) more alive!

Every time I do my moving and breathing, I can feel this unity and also the consciousness of being part of this wonder we call life. I get also quiet inside, and I can feel that it acts very positive to my health. My cells love to get fresh air. Sometimes I do my practice in nature, which is as powerful as a church.

Your Seven-Minute Wonder is your time to care for yourself. By doing it every day, the movements will become more natural, and the process will require less thought—the wisdom of your body and breath will learn to move together as a seamless process. As your practice matures, it will become an exquisite pleasure that allows strength and receptivity to blossom and grow.

You are totally supported by the nurturing force of life. Your practice is a gentle reminder that there is no requirement to be anything other than that which you already are.

Jackie Sherman, Professor of Nursing

When I wake up in the morning, before dawn, usually from a feeling of anxiety instead of by the sound of the alarm clock, I look forward to my seven minutes of moving and breathing. This is a time when no one can get me, or interrupt me, and I have the opportunity to center myself before moving on with my day as a nursing professor at a California university. The anxiety I wake up to has usually subsided after those precious seven minutes of practice.

For years I believed that I needed to attend a ninety-minute exercise class in order to receive this kind of benefit. Now I realize that this isn't so. In fact, being alone with my breath and movement wherever it takes me is more effective than attending a class, which is geared to the masses and not the individual. Who knows us better than we know ourselves? My breath is my guide and dear friend. I obey my breath each day.

Finally, your inherent bodily intimacy is what it's all about. This reveals everything! As with anything in life that you value and believe in, it is important that you set a clear intention to do your practice and continue on the path with continuity and certainty. Once you have mastered the breath and movement sequences, they become a resource that you can take with you wherever you go. As long as you can breathe, you can do your practice. After you do your practice, you may use this reflection:

Love Flows

You are a flower blooming in your own garden. The beauty of each individual person has blossomed into life just as an exquisite and intricate flower shimmers into bloom. As the petals of a lotus flower slowly unfurl in perfect form, you unfold in all directions as a beautiful life. Beginning at conception, the heart, the first cell of life, multiplies to become the whole body. The heart is in every cell. The whole body is the heart. And the whole body is the lotus in full bloom.

The connection between the unseen Source, nurturing force, and body can be felt as a lotus in bloom. The heart arises from the male-female union, and continues to give and receive the masculine and feminine qualities of life. Life is the exact surrender of male and female to each other that allows the nurturing flow. The whole body is the temple from which the heart is shining. The heart is where left merges with right, above with below, front with back, inhale with exhale, outer with inner, female with male, strength with receptivity. It's where heaven meets earth and spirit takes form. The heart resides in a depth and location that cannot be intentionally or willfully discovered but is felt naturally when the whole body is relaxed and participating in its life and relationships.

When your mother and father surrendered to each other, one cell of life appeared. Spirit took form, and from the source to a tangible reality, you grew as life. Within a matter of seconds, minutes, hours, days, months, the beauty of life flowered like an astonishing bright blossom. When you rest at the tip of its petals, in your own skin and in the intimacy of your ordinary condi-

tion and relationships, Nurturing Source energy moves from the heart through your whole body into all natural relatedness. This nurturing source moves through all things. It is at once mental, physical, spiritual, sexual, and cosmic. It is the energetic current of life, the Source, the live wire of existence that continually rolls through you and everything on earth.

These energetic elements move and fluctuate all around you but have a direct line to the heart. Knowing this is ultimate intimacy. It connects heaven and earth, links your body to the stars and your toes to the Divine. If you want to experience it, surrender to your whole body, to your breath, to your relationships—to all ordinary experience. The heart will flow. It is flowing and flowering. Traditionally visualized as a lotus with eight petals, the heart center sends out vital energy into the crown above and down to the base of the body and spinal column, left to right and diagonally. Visualize the lotus flower in bloom in your heart to remind yourself that you are the sheer wonder, beauty, and intelligence of life.

This visual image of a flower in full bloom from your heart is an anciently given form of Nurturing Source Reality—the essence of all life that some call God—that appears as your own form and the wonder of your life. Each petal is known to have a particular life function or power that it gives to you as it unfolds, becoming your embodiment. At the end of the Promise practice, it will be appropriate for many to include their own cultural practices, such as prayer, *puja*, liturgy, chant, or any ritual that is familiar and meaningful to you. I can promise you that the Promise Practice will empower your cultural forms. These practices are the very means by which cultural ideals can become true for you. In the ancient world, the Promise was known as *sadhana* (from an ancient root word meaning "to succeed or attain"), signifying that which you actually *can* do—that is, the practical means to actualize your inspiration.

I have seen friends of the Muslim, Christian, Buddhist, Hindu, and Jewish faiths all able to connect deeply to the visions of their belief systems through the Promise Practice. It reveals the commonality of all human faiths, while celebrating their wonderful differences. In chapter 4, I referred to a group of Islamic women who, through doing the Promise, found the depth of their great culture of love, while their Jewish neighbors also were heartened by their practice—in both case, amidst difficult circumstances. Both cultures were able to share their differences and unite through their practice, which is inclusive of all diversity.

So now merge with your god, your guru, your avatar, your deity, your ancestors, your mountain, your river, your ocean, your life. There is no need for seeking, because your union with these forms of reality is already in place.

The Science of the Promise

I had the good fortune to teach the Promise to Dr. Rosalie Chapple, who trained in anatomy and physiology and holds a PhD in animal physiology from the University of

Sydney. Dr. Chapple now teaches environmental sustainability and ecosystem management at the Institute of Environmental Studies at the University of New South Wales in Sydney. But she has also been an avid practitioner of the Promise for over twenty years and believes, as she told me, "If we all practiced the Promise, I think we'd develop a sustainable society."

After Rosalie had absorbed the principles of the Promise in her daily practice, I wondered if she could apply her academic knowledge and experience to the underlying neurophysiology of it. That's a technical way of saying that all the things I've been telling you about the benefits of breathing slowly and rhythmically, and connecting breath movement with slow, rhythmic body movements, actually have a basis in science. Indeed, scientific studies about the benefits of certain kinds of breathing and movement date back to the middle of the last century at least. But since there have been no clinical studies of the Promise per se, I asked Dr. Chapple if she could put her experience into terms that would reflect the outcomes of previous studies, in language that everyone can understand. Here is what she wrote:

The Physical and Mental Health Benefits of the Promise
ROSALIE CHAPPLE, PhD

The Promise Practice can be seen as a holistic neurophysiological workout. By that I mean it works on the whole system, and has benefits for just about every physical process of the body and mind. The simple control of breath helps us in becoming more resilient to stress. As we have been told before, stress is the biggest killer, and so our management of this epidemic condition offers a host of other benefits.

More and more scientific studies confirm that the mind-body interventions derived from this kind of practice (including the breathing, physical postures, and visualization) alleviate many stress-related mental and physical disorders. Some of these physical conditions are:

- Asthma
- High blood pressure
- Cardiac illness
- Elevated cholesterol
- Irritable bowel syndrome
- Insomnia
- Multiple sclerosis
- Fibromyalgia
- Epilepsy
- Rheumatoid arthritis
- Dysmenorrhea

When we are doing the practice, we bring down the heart rate, which tells the body to relax at all levels. Other benefits of the practice are less obvious but have a greatly positive impact on overall health and well-being. In particular, the practice is a powerful remedy to a variety of mental health conditions. There is reliable clinical evidence for the use of moving and breathing in the treatment of depression, anxiety, and post-traumatic stress disorder.

Control and regulation of the breath is the most important part of the practice. Breathing is controlled by both voluntary and involuntary mechanisms, with complex neuroendocrine feedback mechanisms. The autonomic nervous system, which has a major role in the body's stress response, is made up of the sympathetic and parasympathetic nervous systems. The sympathetic nervous system accelerates the heartbeat, inhibits indigestion, and stimulates the release of the hormone adrenaline (also known as epinephrine). It mediates the fight-or-flight response: the biological response of animals and humans to acute stress that prepares the body for immediate action. The parasympathetic nervous system helps bring the body back into balance by inducing the relaxation response, which slows the heartbeat and stimulates digestion.

Modern lifestyles are commonly associated with chronic stress. When we are working to meet an impossible deadline, it is like your "accelerator" is being floored constantly. High levels of adrenaline are driving us, which often leads to a myriad of health problems, such as heart disease. A common treatment for heart problems is the use of beta-blockers, which are drugs that impede the fight-or-flight response. The impact of the Promise Practice on the neuroendocrine system and the relaxation response means that it can provide a simple and readily available practice to guard against health problems such as heart disease. Deliberate control of the breath helps to modulate autonomic nervous system functions. Slow breathing with prolonged expiration physically reduces anxiety. The reduction of sympathetic activity and the overall increase in parasympathetic nervous system tone is integral to the therapeutic actions listed above.

Dr. Rosalie Chapple: The Science of Love and Intimacy

As the Promise shows, the regular and sustained practice of breath and body movement leads to an increased level of intimacy. There is a direct physiological basis for this. Increased depth of breathing enlivens the body and mind at a cellular level, and we find that empathic response and heightened connection to other people results. Further, studies of cardiovascular health have shown a correlation between increased blood flow and increases in libido and sexual function. This reduces the requirement for mechanical or pharmaceutical interventions that have become the norm in maintaining sexual activity, especially in men as they age. Sexual functioning in general is optimized when the cardiovascular system is functioning well. Intimacy with the body and breath brings about intimacy with others.

CHAPTER 15

Meditation Gone Mad

*There is nothing to attain! It is the search, the seeking,
that is the problem. It is like looking for your glasses
when they are already on your head.*

To those of you who have some background in
meditation, the practices presented in this book might
seem new or unusual. Conventional meditation practice
often creates a kind of dissociation between regular life
and meditative life. You may not be aware of this barrier,
but it can, in some cases, create conflict or serious problems in your life—even though that is often the very thing
you were seeking to resolve!

The kind of meditation that arises from doing Your
Seven-Minute Wonder is immediately fruitful. It comes
about not by "witnessing" the world as an object but
through merging *with* your experience and thoroughly
embracing your world.

Natural meditation arises from intimate connection
with all ordinary conditions. It is clarity of mind, intimately connected to what is. It is not an attempt to become

something, or to get somewhere as if we are not already somewhere. It should be easy, because we are *already* intimate with our life. It's not about stepping away from life and residing as awareness, the common understanding of meditation derived from Buddhism, now popularized even in the mental health model of "stress reduction."

Gautama Buddha was experienced in the Promise meditation, and so was Jesus! They were in the natural state of "mind fullness," an absorption in *all* experience, not in the dissociated "mindfulness" of residing as an outside, detached witness—a doctrinal idea invented hundreds of years later in an all-male Buddhist order. That Jesus was a Promise meditator is revealed in his advice to "love thy neighbor as thyself." Indeed, the idea of celibacy and monastic renunciation came to both doctrines hundreds of years after the lives of the key founders. Clearly, their lives and instruction imply the *embracing of all* your experiences and not just witnessing them!

This embrace of life, realized by the Buddha and by Jesus, allows you to feel your true nature, reality itself, or Real God. Over time, however, this spiritual sublimity was converted into abstract ideals and given quite another frame. The original experience of meditation was lost. Humanity had its intimacy taken away. In the ancient world, meditative practices arose in this context of intimate connection with life. Moving and breathing, and relationships of all kinds, were inherent to the life of meditation. This connection was believed to be the very method by which the mind becomes clear, and by which deep awareness of the source or substance of all experience arises. When it becomes obvious to a practitioner that there is *only* the Heart, or God, then meditation never creates dissociation from our actual experience. Only through that experience—embodied and visceral—did anyone realize Source Reality in the first place!

As I've said before, if you're searching for God, it implies that God does not already exist as part of you, and so it follows that if you're using meditation as a tool in this futile search, you're bound to be frustrated. That is why I say the universal method and meditation of all wisdom culture is enjoyment of the actual embodied love relationship between two people.

And if meditation itself is a distant state you're trying to reach, this will add to your frustration. When you *try* to meditate, you just get good at *trying to meditate,* but *not* at actually meditating itself. It's like sleeping: the more you try to sleep, the more restless and unable to sleep you become. You are more likely to fall asleep if you have created the conditions for it to come about. Once your basic needs have been attended to—you're tired, comfortable, warm, and have the lights out—you fall asleep naturally.

It's the same with meditation. Create the right conditions, and meditation will naturally and easily arise. Here is where Your Seven-Minute Wonder will help you. The intimacy of breath and movement, especially when it becomes a daily routine, gives rise to meditation. Trying to meditate without this practice is tantamount to trying to sleep while standing up, with all the lights on.

The Promise Practice, meditation, and life are a seamless process. It clears the mind and allows for intimate connection of every kind, including the Source of all. Many experienced meditation practitioners will find that the Promise enhances what they have already been taught, but it also provides them with a practice to integrate their experience into the ordinary conditions of life. It's a powerful tool.

Puay's Story:
Anyone Who Can Breathe Can Practice

Puay, a Buddhist teacher from Singapore, learned the Promise after having spent many years devoted to meditation practice. He then attended a traditional Buddhist meditation retreat held at a monastery:

Attending the retreat, I had the quiet space to contemplate on what I felt earlier was a conflict between the Promise message and the Buddha's teachings. Being a relatively new student of Buddha's teachings, I make the crucial distinction between what the Buddha taught and Buddhism, the latter being a religion where humans have reinterpreted certain propositions of facts to be believed in. To me, belief systems are dogmatic and separatist. That is, those who believe certain sets of propositions that claim to be true become "Buddhists." Buddhists are then distinguished from Christians, Muslims, Hindus, Jews, and others who believe different sets of propositions.

But the Buddha's teachings are relevant to all who are connected to their breath—what the Promise teaches—not things to believe in but situations that suggest a course of inquiry, testing, and experiencing. I started to realize that the Promise is actually teaching what the Buddha taught! For instance, the Buddha taught that wanting something is a grasping; a clinging. It is this attachment that brings about misery, for grasping creates the mismatch between the now and "if only." The Buddha also taught that meditation is not a physical posture (for example, what is prevalent in many "meditation" centers, in which "meditators" assume the lotus position, "doing" seated meditation) but a mental posture—an awareness of here and now.

In the middle of one class, the monk teacher invited me to take over the role of teaching the Promise to the students every morning. There were about fifty of them, mostly devout Buddhists practicing seated "meditation," hoping to achieve something beyond the pain in their knees, their back, and their head. Some raised their arms to ask if they could "do" the Promise in their conditions. I reassured them that anyone who can breathe can practice. I also asked for their open-mindedness. The next morning before dawn, the crowd gathered again, and I decided to proceed with my cheeky plan. I told everyone, "Uh, no meditation this morning. I changed my mind. We shall get intimate instead."

Then there was awkward silence. I glanced at the monk. He had a soft smile, which I took to mean, "Go ahead, strut your stuff."

I continued, "Shall we get intimate now?" Some stopped breathing, I think. And I added, "With our breath? As our lover." There was some laughter at the back. Others were still confused, wanting out. Over the days, we progressed to taking our lover (the breath) on a tour of the body, inhaling so thoroughly, just like we do before we kiss our lover. We moved on to embracing our lover and not wanting him/her to change in any way, *to having the first fight with our beloved. Most important, the monastery was fine with it. For it is what the Buddha taught. The Promise brought new joy and life into the meditation we had always loved.*

As Puay's story shows, the practice of breath and movement actually deepens rather than undermines any experience of meditation. There is no conflict here, just a wonderful opportunity to bring about greater peace and power through the intimate union of opposites within the body. A physical process of moving the body in unison with the breath naturally creates the ideal circumstances for a meditative state to arise. By aiding the flow of the breath in your body with appropriate movements, you can begin to participate in and nurture a state of integration and harmony that naturally precedes a condition of peace and stillness.

Our natural state is one of peace and power, and the basis on which our fundamental existence rests. We share this not only with each other but also with the oceans, mountains, suns, moons, and stars as the underlying, unifying force of all reality. In order to access it, we need not cultivate anything but simply allow these qualities to flourish as our obvious innate perfection.

Mary's Story:
Meditating Without Even Trying

(Mary is our Irish farmer friend, from whom we heard earlier.)

After taking a workshop in which I was told that I didn't have to try to meditate, I felt relief as a huge self-burden lifted off my back. The next thing I knew, I was meditating without even trying. Then I was encouraged to just do my seven minutes of moving and breathing each day and see how I felt. I took up this suggestion, and have been honestly more balanced and centered ever since. There is power in consciously being aware of your own inhale and exhale and the union it creates with yourself. I am a huge believer that everyone would benefit from a simple seven minutes of this daily practice. There is no doubt in my mind that we would see tremendous positive transformations in people and our world.

In order for meditation to arise, you need to let go of any previously held concepts of it as an actively attainable state that requires exacting postures, heroic acts of mind control, or weeklong silent retreats to master. What you can do instead is your daily seven minutes of moving the body in unison with the breath. By aiding the movement of the breath in the body with appropriate movements, you can participate in a state of integration and harmony that naturally precedes a condition of peace and stillness. We cannot meditate actively. What we can do is cultivate fertile ground in which the seeds of meditation will begin to blossom and grow.

Stop Looking

It is important to remember that you are not engaging in this process in preparation for some future realization or higher reality but as a participation in your own fundamental reality already given. A meditative state may arise as a result of this, or it may not. At the end of your practice, you may feel compelled to rest in the stillness that comes about, but it is not something that is forced or that you need to impose on yourself.

Even if you don't feel a tangible result all of the time, you must continue to practice. With this practice, you will spontaneously and unpredictably feel your direct connection to life and involve yourself in a daily ritual of intimacy. Please inquire into every way that you seek for something other than what you *are*. You can even use the phrase "Stop looking" like a gentle mantra, as an instruction for the mind as you inspect every kind of mental structure of seeking that has been put in you, and allow them to dissolve in the feelings of intimate connection to all that is. If you use traditional cultural meditations, such as your relationship with your teacher, Avatar, sacred places, or objects of intimacy, you are already at one with them, and no seeking is required.

As you move through your practice, do not search for any mind-blowing experience; or seek conditions or circumstances that you may have read about or been told about; or that you may have felt in the past on that one sublime day when everything was perfect. People often attend a retreat or a meditation workshop and manage to experience a kind of blissful state. It may have to do with the location in lovely countryside, or being surrounded by a group of like-minded souls. Then they return home, to the city, or to their job, or to the challenges of raising a family, or to living a relationship, and they wonder why they can't meditate the way they did during the retreat. To return to the metaphor of falling asleep, it's like remembering how well you slept after you spent the day in your garden or hiking the mountains, or doing satisfying work when you felt in the zone. When your head hit the pillow, you fell asleep effortlessly. Then there are days when you don't get any exercise, or feel trapped by your job or under financial or emotional pressures. To compensate for the stress, you eat a huge meal and watch hours of television—and then you wonder why you can't fall asleep, and just toss and turn all night.

So practice naturally, daily, but not obsessively, no matter how good or bad you feel. You make natural beneficial life changes as you go along. Don't worry that you aren't spending hours trying to meditate and not getting any results. There is no need to look for anything. Source or God is not absent. The Promise not only facilitates meditation, it *is* meditation.

Just continue with your intimate practice of body, breath, and relationship, in that order. Allow for the full range of experience to flourish. You will feel your gracefull life and enjoy it as it is now, at this very moment. Stop looking. Start living your wonder-full life.

CHAPTER 16

A Soft Message for a Hard Time

Human contentment, wellness, and wisdom are in the power of opposites in union: left to right, above to below, inhalation to exhalation, strength to receptivity, within to without, man to woman—the very means by which source becomes seen and spirit takes form in the nurturing force of life.

AT THE TIME OF THE SEPTEMBER 11, 2001, DISASTERS at the World Trade Center in New York City, I lived two blocks away on South End Avenue. Our apartment building was trashed. That morning, my wife had caught the train beneath the Twin Towers two minutes before the first plane hit. She came up from the subway a short time later to experience the horror of the towers ablaze. The sickening stench of plastic, concrete, and flesh lingered for months, and our apartment was unlivable, cracked and covered with thick, deathly ash. Our lives were turned upside down. Really, the life of the whole planet has been turned upside down through the ignorance of those who believe that a higher reality exists, dissociated from life on earth.

209

Since the beginning of recorded history, we have observed this abuse of one another. Once we developed the power of meaning, the ability to abstract from the physical, we dissociated ourselves from the natural state. Some believe that the development of alphabets composed of abstract symbols rewired the human brain, shifting our dominant focus from the intuitive, spatial right brain to the more logical, literal left brain. This further dissociates us from our natural state, the Nurturing Source of all life, and results in the aberrant behavior of humanity. For example, we are the only species that systematically kills its own kind.

It is time to return to what is natural, to protect ourselves, one another, and nature Herself, our great nurturing source. Then we will make good use of our wonderful abilities of abstraction, meaning, science, and technology. These will serve our intimacy, our sacred reality, instead of reinforcing an imagined separation and fear.

Many of us feel overwhelmed by the endless traumas that the daily news announces. The evolution into our natural state seems to make us only more vulnerable to others' pain. I maintain that this is as it should be. It is only natural to feel anger and pain so that we are moved to take action. Strong individuals, leaders, and nations have a special responsibility to make the change. But as in all things, that strength must become receptive. We need "inspiration": to breathe in and let strength give space for the air to come in; for grace to come down on us. Just as strength is receiving in the cycles of inhalation and exhalation of the Promise Practice, male strength has a special responsibility to receive his feminine counterpart, not merely possess or control her. The ultimate politics is the democracy of male-female equality and mutual coopera- tion. When we cooperate with what is natural, the peace and power of the natural state will come through us.

This is a particular responsibility of men, because strength must receive life to survive; otherwise it destroys itself. The control of the feminine and abuse of the natural state over many generations is finally being addressed in personal and public life. Our sex will be healed and made entirely positive. Then we will know peace on earth.

With all that in mind, I made myself available to teach the Promise in the midst of the dreadful trauma of down- town Manhattan. Subsequently, because my teaching schedule carries me across the globe, I have made contact among the devastated lives of the endless Middle East wars and the Arab Spring, and I also witnessed the natural disasters of the earthquakes of New Zealand and Japan in 2011. In every case, I have seen how, even in the midst of terrible difficulty, comfort and help are given by life itself. Given by breath, given by one another in the pas- sion of nurturing friendship. There is enormous power in this simple practice that gives comfort, stress release, and healing. When the chips are down, when we seem to be beyond hope, the best of human nature kicks in. After New Zealand and Japan were struck by earthquakes within a few weeks, both countries put many caring boots on each other's ground within twenty-four hours. Our natural need is to protect and care for one another and allow the nurturing force of reality to flow through us all.

Gail Mondry's Story:
The New York Tragedy

Thirty days after the tragedy of 9/11, I traveled to Manhattan with my husband for a fund-raising seminar. I remember being quite frightened by all the security in the airports and swept up in the paranoia as security dumped out my Yoga mat bag to see what I was really carrying into New York. Because my husband would be involved in meetings all day, I wanted to ease my mind, and was drawn to a daylong Promise intensive, which was being offered at a studio downtown.

Emerging from the subway, I was startled by the astringent smell and the still-visible soot that covered every surface. When I walked into the studio, almost one hunded very nervous teachers were grabbing bolsters, blocks, straps, and a space on the floor as they do in regular Yoga fitness classes. I had never used props, but I started to grab for them too, as I got caught up in the climate of the room. Nervous chatter filled the studio until our teacher flowed in.

Throughout the day, we never touched a strap, block, or bolster. Instead of simply pushing through our anxieties, we were gently shown how to come back to the intimacy of our breath, to touch our hearts, our inner body of wisdom. Our teacher narrowed our focus to more present and physical actions: breathing and moving, focused and peaceful in a flow of life that nurtured us. We were no longer daunted by distant events. I was forever changed as a practitioner and teacher by the Promise I learned that day in the shadow of devastation, and left that workshop a more grounded and hopeful person. Mark has always taught from his heart and his authentic upbringing, but for me, receiving it as a visceral experience so close to ground zero was the "aha" moment of a growing teacher.

The Challenge of Depression

A practical course of action is necessary if we wish to lift ourselves out of unwanted situations or circumstances. No change will come about with a blinding flash of light, but rather with a slow, steady progression from day to day. Here is where a daily practice can be helpful and effective. And if it's simple and can be done in a short period of time, it is likely to be maintained. It is the maintaining of the practice—the repetition and the routine—that will bring about long-term benefits and healing.

Lucy's Story:
Wanting to Avoid All Feeling

Lucy has been a nurse for over thirty years, taking care of other people mainly in their own homes. Like many caregivers, though, she hasn't always taken good care of herself. Although Lucy worked full-time for much of her career, she was usually paid per diem, meaning that she could make up her own schedule. As long as she saw the patients she was assigned, she could do so at her own pace, and she enjoyed that freedom. Then she took a job as a nursing supervisor, because it offered a better salary and health benefits for her family. But now she had to be in the office every day from eight thirty until five o'clock, with only two weeks of vacation each year. After several years, the inflexible schedule and lack of personal freedom started to make her feel depressed. She also grew less active and started to gain weight, which made her feel even more depressed. Here is how Lucy tells it:

I admit that I'm a couch potato and a depressive. I have always shunned sports, although I do like walking and bike riding. As I got older, my activity level dropped, and when my work became more sedentary, I really started putting on weight. My husband is just the opposite, taking long daily walks, cross-country skiing in winter, and working out in his home gym. He wanted me to share his enjoyment of physical exercise and help me keep in shape. First he tried to get me to go skiing, but I was so uncoordinated that I had to drink a little brandy to get over my fear of falling and breaking my leg, even when I skied at a snail's pace! On the few occasions when I tried to join him for a walk, I would have to turn back after just five or ten minutes because I was out of breath.

So when he said he wanted me to join him in something called Your Seven-Minute Wonder, I thought, "Great, here we go again. Another Bataan Death March!" He tried to accommodate me, fearing that I would lose interest—like I usually do in all activities that involve physical exertion—and agreed to do it in the mornings, when I felt most energetic. I got out my aqua-colored exercise mat that I had not used for years, because the thought of putting on a Yoga or Tae Bo DVD was overwhelming. But the first day, I just followed him through the practice, enjoy-

ing it without any sense of pressure. I noticed the blue sky and winter trees outside my window. And then it was over before I knew it. I was able to complete the practice without any feelings of dread or boredom. That is what strikes me the most about the Promise: I am not bored by this exercise.

My husband kept telling me to pay attention to my breathing, but my breath was the last thing I noticed. That was unusual, because I have asthma and usually have trouble breathing when I exercise. But the slow, rhythmic movements combined body and breath in a way that seemed effortless.

I liked that he called this practice the Promise, and that I was supposed to promise to do it every day for forty days and see what happened. Some mornings it would be difficult for me—not because it was physically stressful but because I was depressed and wanting to avoid all feeling. But I remembered my commitment to the Promise and forced myself to do it. One day I felt anxiety, and halfway through just wanted to scream and stop. Then I realized that was because I wanted to stop feeling and being alive. But this practice calls you back to your center. Once I started doing it, I felt grounded. I may have had the same problems, but I was able to notice the trees outside the window. I also noticed how much my breath is involved in maintaining my emotional state.

As someone who works in the public health field, I can't help thinking that the Promise could help so many ordinary people cope with depression and weight gain resulting from inactivity. Because it's easy to learn and doesn't place stress on the joints, even people who are overweight or suffer from asthma can do it on a daily basis.

The Challenge of Addiction

We live in a society of addiction. Fake desires are created and pushed on us in the guise of spiritual or self-improvement ideals, and we do not learn to recognize or act on our real desires. Trying to be something you are not is the cause of human suffering. This is addiction. From the ultimate pop star to a homeless person, we are trying to get somewhere as if we are not already the unadorned marvel of life. The solutions to our plight are usually more of the same: one stronger pill after the other, one exaggeration after the next, as despair increases. Society is on trial. We do not know how to care for even our great artists, let alone the sizable portion of the earth's billions who go to bed hungry each night! We must intervene with our friends and family and let them feel the love that beats their own heart, as life intends. Enable them to find the peace in their connections and directions that work for them. Starting with body and breath!

Life is perfection, but how we live has been a crippling compromise. All over the world, people are claiming their own lives and shrugging off oppressive power structures of every kind. It is a wonderful turnaround. Now let's really give them their own life.

Simone King, a widow and the mother of three beautiful boys, speaks about addiction and sobriety:

I began practicing the Promise at twenty-four and got sober a year later. I had a long period of sobriety filled with life, fam-

ily, and love. When my husband died suddenly, all of this was shattered. He was my best friend, my lover, my coparent, and my biggest fan. It seemed like my relapsing was inevitable. Unfortunately, it took me to a darker place than I could have ever imagined.

I am deeply grateful that Mark came into my life. He saw the most embarrassing details of a desperate life of drinking! In the midst of this, he showed me the practice he refers to as strength receiving. As a single mother with three young sons, I had grown to believe I had to be very strong. I owned businesses, managed staff, and "handled" a huge life of stress. I was really good at this strength part but out of touch with any ability to receive. I was so busy trying to be strong, to survive, that I forgot how to be intimate, with myself, my sons, my staff, my friends, and life itself.

The Promise gave all of that back to me. It began to give me what I was trying to feel in the bottle! This has proven to be abundantly true. I know it can be so for you too. Breathing creates intimacy with body, breath, and life, and out of that intimacy arises the ability to honestly touch and know another human being. These are the greatest gifts life has to offer. This simple program allows you to develop a personal life of everyday intimacy that replaces the desperate attempt to find comfort in addictions. It is too good an opportunity to pass up.

Whatever is going down, even in the midst of financial and family worries, always find time to keep your Promise. There is a wealth in here that money can't buy, and it gives you the treasures of life. You will feel completely loved and nurtured even if social conditions are suggesting otherwise.

CHAPTER 17

Now, Begin! Start Where You Are: Male-Female Union and the Source of Both

Let the wonder and utter connection to life be sufficient. Let breath be sufficient. Let this sitting here be sufficient. Let this reality be sufficient. And start to enjoy the inherent, intrinsic, inborn powers of life that move in us.

As we saw in chapter 8, the continuity of life relies on the attraction of opposites. Life as we know it is a fusion of left and right, above and below, seen and unseen, heaven and earth, male and female, and inhale to exhale. The masculine and feminine forces of life are constantly moving together in an energetic dance that we participate in from birth up to the point when we become mothers and fathers ourselves, and they blend. All creation comes to form through the absolute surrender of the masculine to the feminine in a universal celebration that is demonstrated viscerally through sex. This coming together is an infinite cycle that creates life and allows for new life to flourish and continue.

The evolution of our physicality from the union of male and female takes place without any conscious manipulation or regard to process on our part. Life simply does what it needs to in order to express this overwhelming effulgence of creativity from which everything is born. These qualities are the blueprint of creation and the basis of everyone as a model of wholeness and perfection.

We cannot and should not wish to escape the reality that we are born attached to our mothers, and remain connected to life throughout the rest of our days. This is not a problem. It is a blessing. Born of our mothers, we are supported unconditionally by the forces of creation. We depend on this utter intimacy with life and our unending connection to this same unseen source.

Beginning with our conception and continuing until our deaths, we are exposed continually to all natural forms of intimacy. We are given a constant stream of beautiful examples of life at work—the most obvious and pertinent being pregnancy and motherhood/fatherhood. The journey of form from a single cell of life to a full and complete human being is a mind-blowing process that is unique in its magnificence.

A tangible awareness of our natural state is our birthright and something that should neither be denied nor awarded. Bear in mind that whatever tangled constructs have arisen from our fearful social mind, in nature nothing exists but perfect union, the one unchanging constant that remains amidst the fluctuations of everyday life.

In order to convert these ideas into some form of practical understanding and feeling, you must start your practice. The action of moving the body in coordination with the breath is the process I've been calling strength receiving. Here a mother of three describes it well.

I had always referred to my state of being pregnant as being "strong soft"—it was a simple way of explaining to others what I felt like when I was pregnant. My usually hard physical body developed a softness that I found wonderful. I still felt strong, but all my "hardness" fell away. Since delivering my last baby two and a half years ago, I hadn't been in touch with this strong/soft feeling.

Then I started practicing the Promise. Now I am exploring it daily in my full-body breathing, in putting my palms together softly, and moving through my postures without effort. I feel all my opposites and their mysterious One source.

To enter into this practice is like making love to all of life; it is as exquisite as that. Not only will this have a profound effect on your own life but also on your relationship with everyone around you, including and especially your intimate partner. That is what living is all about: the intimate connection between you and the world.

Juliana Monin, a dancer and teacher from Oakland, California, describes this:

The entry point for me has been the logic of the practice, in which the descending inhale/ascending exhale is described as a technology of love. That idea was something I could easily grasp. It just has made sense to me from the beginning. If I am doing a participatory practice with the polarities that make up life, then I myself must embody those polarities. This understanding, just as an understanding, has given me permission to have my life. I embody those polarities without the practice at all—that is, I come from my mother and father, therefore I am female/male—so the practice gets to be my full-bodied expression and experience of that understanding.

It has occurred to me that regardless of my current physical or psychological or emotional state, when my whole body receives and gives (inhalation/exhalation) in repetition in its continuous cycle, like a heartbeat, my whole body is put in the condition of love. To love is to give and receive, and this practice puts me "in love"! The feeling of love is for me a process, a movement, not a fixed point to be captured. So this whole body loving, allowed by the feeling of belonging to the universe, then lets me give myself to the universe. Every breath now becomes my primary communication between my inner and outer worlds.

I now completely get how we, in our material forms, do feel the infinite, and how the vibrations of the cosmos do take form in our spines. I admit I have resisted my whole life to feel the depth of my power, my worth, and my beauty. This practice has catapulted my personal life and my professional life in dance, as I have more and more been able to trust my experiences and my impulses, and have gone from a proficient dancer-imitator to an actual dancer. This gift of getting to know my movement, my dance, is absolutely priceless.

Finally, it is impossible to speak of a practice of intimacy and *self-love without the mention of sex. Even though my friends sometimes laugh at the idea, I continue insisting that there is nothing more erotic than the private love affair going on inside us. To feel exhalation penetrating and receiving inhalation, and vice versa, and to fully feel the awakening of my spine, have completely brought me into my sexuality, and move me away from the shame, embarrassment, fear, and pain that has surrounded it for so long. I feel "turned on" in all interpretations of that phrase. I knew what John Lennon meant when he sang about how it turned him on that the world is round. I am with you, man!*

I have come to understand that this practice, rather than being about trying to open my heart, is about revealing my already open heart and letting it express through me. It is the stubborn refusal to be shut down and hardened, to dissociate and detach. I just get to be in love. And isn't that what we all want anyway?

Jennifer Patterson's Story: The Hair and Now

Jennifer Patterson is a writer from New York City who had attended a seminar on the Promise. When I met her again a few months later, she was excited to explain to me how she had completely stopped struggling and trying to control her life. She told me that after the seminar, even her hair went into its natural form, and all her friends and family told her how beautiful and natural her hair and she looked. We both laughed a lot.

Like most women I know, I spent the majority of my adult life wrestling with a deeply embedded sense that I was simultaneously not enough (not pretty enough, strong enough, successful enough, thin enough, funny enough) and too much (too honest, too unruly, too ordinary, too wild, too intense). Trying to find my balance under the weight of this polarizing self-image, I spent years "efforting" my way through my life, carefully patrolling and correcting my body, diet, emotions, and even my hair—which is neither fully straight nor fully curly but something in between: fickle, rebellious, and completely unpredictable. That unruly hair of mine needed to be tamed, needed to be smaller, less wild. Like my body. Like my emotions. Every desire, every impulse, every square inch was suspect; a potential enemy in my quest for perfection. Whether executing a perfect Yoga pose or the perfect pose of "woman," my experience in my own body and breath had been hijacked by a self-loathing that is so brilliantly and insidiously peddled to us under the banners of everything from Yoga to couture. The underlying message is that who and what you are is not enough as is. Yet some part of me—some holy, whole, perfect part of me—continued to rebel against the effort, the struggle, the quest. Like my hair, it just couldn't be tamed.

Then I learned the Promise Practice, the essence of which is simply this: you are and have always been enough, and who you are is fully supported and loved in this world. I breathed into that understanding—gave it some room—and for the first time, I moved through a practice completely in my body, no longer wrestling with or against it but simply savoring each breath as it met and nourished the fabric of my body. I was at peace.

And silly as it may sound, my hair changed too. Or, more

precisely, I surrendered and embraced my hair and stopped fighting to control, tame, or change it. People commented on how great I looked, asking if I had done something different, and my response was often, "No, I just stopped doing." I had settled back and found rest in who I am and what I am. But when I say that even my hair changed, I am not saying that I left it unattended or dismissed it as somehow lowly or superficial. I didn't transcend my hair. No, I play with my hair and enjoy its quirky, totally unpredictable nature. The difference is that I don't fight to make it something it isn't. I participate with my hair—and the everyday ordinariness of it, my job, my family, my emotions, my thoughts, and my life as extraordinary articulations of the Divine itself. Not too much, and always enough. "Seriously but not humorlessly!" as Mark would remind me.

CHAPTER 18

Bringing It All Back Home

The Promise is a literal promise to yourself and to me to practice daily Your Seven-Minute Wonder. It is an interwoven promise. You Promise to keep your promise, and I promise you wonderful results.

OFTEN WHEN WE LEARN SOMETHING NEW, IT TAKES some time to fully absorb all the information and adapt it into our experiences. Many of the ideas that I have shared with you in the Promise may be new to you and give you cause for some reflection. This is perfectly okay, and you should feel relaxed about taking some time to digest what has been discussed. The myths that have been handed down to us by society and traditional religious doctrine are deeply embedded, and so for many of you, this book will herald the start of a new perspective. Rest assured that all the wisdom in this book has been passed down directly to me by my teachers, who are profound scholars, not businessmen!

I took it on myself and adapted it from my own background and insights. I then adapted it to the needs of thousands of people who now have "gotten it." They all became my teachers and made this delivery possible. It is possible to "get it" all at once and practice it. A long effort of heroic practice and arduous learning is not required, as if there were a future ideal to attain. Just practice steadily in the way that is right for you. What I have shared with you will be of vast benefit to you in your life, as well as all those with whom you are in relationship. The depth of this knowledge is vast, and there are certain major points that I want to make clear to you now, so that at any time you may refer to this chapter to review the key messages of the Promise. We have already prepared your study notes.

The Promise Principles

The Promise Practice is *direct* intimacy with the *given* reality that is nothing other than nurturing, regeneration, and continuity. It must be adapted to your unique differences, body type, age, health, lifestyle, and culture. It is a catalyst for you to realize all your potential in all relations, with health, love, sex, career, money, creativity, and the Source of all.

- *You* are the extreme intelligence of life. If there is such a thing as an unseen Source, it is appearing as this wonder that is you.

- Nurturing Source Reality is present in you, *as you,* the utter uniqueness that is you. In your intimacy with all ordinary conditions, you are nurtured and will know the natural state, reality itself.

- The Promise Practice is participation in the union of all opposites. It reveals the source of all opposites known in the traditions as the heart, nurturing source, or God, reality itself. "The two" become One, while remaining two, differentiated, and wholly unique. The Promise gives you direct union to the anciently promised heart while you remain completely autonomous and individuated. It delivers the promise.

- The Promise enables you to tangibly experience abstract ideals in your inherent Oneness with life, which is everyOne's intrinsic condition and birthright. The practice is necessary to dissolve the false dichotomy between the knowledge holder, the teacher, and the seeker in the great mutual affection and the One Reality of all.

- Doctrines, as power structures of many kinds, have embedded in us the presumption that we need to seek for some higher self or alternative state—to know God as a future possibility, for example. Rest assured that this is not the case. In fact, the answer you seek is already here. You can radically stop searching now and abide as you are. The looking is the problem that implies the absence of what you seek. Searching for what you already are, or trying to be something that you are not, is human suffering. This has been put in you like a virus or defective software. The body throws it out once it is recognized, and restores itself to the natural state. This may occur suddenly, like an explosion of unobstructed life from within, or in a gradual restoration of intimate connection to reality.

• There is no need to seek anything. The one who seeks is a socially constructed identity that has no basis in reality. All there is, is reality—and you are that. You are already all that you need. Everything you want is provided, so embrace all aspects of life. Just as we do not seek for the sun, but enjoy the sun, so we do not need to seek for our Source. We enjoy what is already given. Spiritual life is not about seeking but about devoted participation in what *is*. Man's heaven has created a hell of this abundant paradise in the denial of the ordinary for imagined higher states. This is now addressed and corrected for you and for future generations.

• Source and the seen are One. Therefore, the seen is full and sufficient. A search for Source by manipulating or denying the seen is not required. The seen is as profound and mysterious as the idea of Source.

• By intimacy with all ordinary seen conditions, Nurturing Source, the natural state of Reality, the Heart, or Real God, is known. Through intimacy with all aspects of life, including breath, body, and relationship, all aspects of the given reality, you will feel your peace and power—not through the denial of the seen.

- Source Reality, the natural state, becomes a certainty for you, as the context of all conditions. This does not cause dissociation from others, from individuality, or from any conditions—because intimacy with all ordinary conditions is the very means by which you realize it. You know all conditions and individuals, including yourself, to be arising in and as reality itself. All "things" may be felt as the visibility and vibration of reality only, and do not imply separation from that.

- The entire development of civilization has been built upon humankind's need to acknowledge special objects, places, people, gurus, deities, and avatars as the embodiment of reality. (Even the nondual traditions such as Vedanta or Buddhism that speak of "no object" or "emptiness" as their philosophy, paradoxically use the link to the "object" of sacred personality, their guru or teacher, as their principal means; and compassion to all "beings" or the flow of nurturing is their essential message.) The Promise Practice ensures that teacher-student relationships are natural, actual, and of mutual affection—not the social dynamic of knower and seeker. The individual is truly empowered in the One Reality, the natural state of the universe. The Promise was not given in the abstract text and the historic expansion of doctrine. Yet it was the origin and practicum; the vital means to realize the abstract ideals of doctrine. Anciently, the Promise Practice was axiomatic; just assumed to be there in the social context. Now it is back and available to all, always and in all ways.

- Pain is an intrinsic function of nature and not the enemy. It is healing, and it facilitates necessary change. Every kind of pain leads you through obstructions to freedom. Understand that pain is an aspect of nurturing force. Allow it to function and do its work. It naturally reduces itself as a quality of its function.

- The Heart is where all opposites originate and return: above and below, left and right, inhalation and exhalation, strength receiving, male and female, within and without. It is where Source becomes seen, or Spirit takes form as you. When the opposites took form as your mother and father, perfectly merged, you arrived. The heart is the first cell of life that blooms as you, the whole body, and all its relationships. It is the source of all nurturing. The flow of nurturing force may be felt as spirals from the heart, like a flower in full bloom to all areas of the body and beyond in all relationships. The heart does not need to be located or concentrated upon but is simply felt when the whole body is integrated in all that is. And it *is*, already given.

- By participating in the union of any or all the opposites, the natural state or Source Reality is known. It is easy, requiring no struggle or heroic effort. Participation in any of the opposites serves all others. We have no choice but to participate in all the opposites. They cannot be bypassed. Sex, the unreserved respect for male-female mutuality, cannot be bypassed in an attempt to know God. It is the very means.

- Exhalation-inhalation, strength that is receptive, is the primary polarity that allows for realization of unobstructed male and female union and the source of both. Each gathers the strength of the other in a nurturing flow. All of life is formed from this strength-receiving formula, just as a great tree has a strong trunk and roots, yet its foliage is soft and receptive, gathering nutrients from above. One aspect depends on the other. This is your own quality, and it is easily felt as the Promise Practice.

- The body is one with its own breath. The body loves its breath just as we love one another in utter connectedness, by which new life comes.

- All this is made possible through actual and natural, nonobsessive, daily practice of the Promise.

- In the Promise Practice, the body movement *is* the breath movement. Allow the breath to start and end each movement. Inhalation is receptivity from above. Exhalation is strength from below. The intelligent cooperation of muscle groups above to below serves the breath in the polarity of strength receiving. The head bows to its source, the heart, while the strength of the base supports the heart. Body, breath, meditation, and life are a seamless process. Clarity of mind, or intimacy that is meditation, arises naturally as a personal power and cannot be practiced willfully, just as sleep comes naturally when conditions are right.

- There *is* no separation. You *are* what you are looking for. The looking creates the imaginary loss. So stop looking, start living. It is intimacy we need, not enlightenment. Yet intimacy gives us everything, including enlightenment.

You may like simply to read these phrases, or, in time, as you develop your own practice, you may find that spontaneous realizations occur. If this happens, you can write them down and add to the principles—your personal Promise Practice and insights. True learning is always an evolving process and is facilitated only by direct experience. Even the oldest sacred texts in the world continue to expand as practitioners experience facets of their truth. The texts of the great Upanishadic tradition across thousands of years, for example, are a continual flow of nurturing, like a great river of wisdom literature from ancient to present time and onward. The Upanishads held the

Promise and the great understandings that became world religion. There is no beginning and no end. The Promise can be your living-and-breathing document and your contribution to the great tradition.

Conversations with My Teacher

The teacher I mentioned back in chapter 1, and whose wisdom I have invoked throughout, said so many marvelous things that they belong in any enumeration of the Promise Principles. Apply them as you see fit.

- The peace you are seeking is already inside you.

- The extraordinary intelligence of the biological organism is all that is necessary for good living.

- If you have the courage to touch life for the first time, you will never know what hit you.

- Real silence is explosive; it is not the dead state of mind that spiritual seekers think. This is volcanic in its nature, bubbling all the time.

- To be yourself requires extraordinary intelligence. You are blessed with that intelligence; nobody need give it to you, nobody can take it away from you. He or she who lets that express itself in its own way is a natural man or woman.

- The mystique of enlightenment is based upon the idea of transforming your self. I maintain that there is nothing to change or transform.

- To be yourself is very easy; you don't have to do a thing. No effort is necessary. You don't have to exercise your will. You don't have to do anything to be yourself. But to be something other than what you are, you have to do a lot of things.

- Man cannot be anything other than what he is.

- You are not one thing and the life another. It is one unitary movement.

- This body doesn't want to learn anything. Left to itself, it has tremendous intelligence.

- The sex experience is the one thing in life you have that comes close to being a firsthand experience, not the grotesque duplication of social patterning.

- When the movement in the direction of becoming something other than what you are isn't there anymore, you are not in conflict with yourself.

- The Natural State is a state of great sensitivity—but this is a physical sensitivity of the senses . . . There is compassion only in the sense that there are no "others" for me, and so there is no separation.

- You have to touch life at a point where nobody has touched it before. Nobody can teach you that.

One Love

Be we Buddhist, Christian, Jewish, Muslim, Hindu, Taoist, Sikh, Rastafarian, atheist, agnostic, secular humanist, or any derivative thereof, all of us everywhere can realize our dreams, ideals, and inspirations with the Promise. I remember teaching a Roman Catholic nun named Sister Cecile in New Zealand. She told me that the Promise had enabled her to feel the depth of her faith and released her from the effort of trying to be a good nun, of trying to get somewhere in her institution's arbitrary spiritual improvement criteria. Further, Sister Cecile reported that she stopped struggling with the Pope when she felt her relationship to God was direct, requiring no mediation. Somehow she came to peace with authority. She said humorously that she had suddenly realized that the patron saint of her religious order was also a Promise practitioner, when she saw a painting of him in nine different postures of prayer. She was so happy.

The Islamic world, too, has something wonderful as it comes together in the great mosques of love to practice whole body prayer. My Muslim friends also say that the Promise has enabled them to feel personally the reality of their faith as they practice their prayer of breath and esoteric union with All, or Allah. Promise practitioners celebrate the obvious commonality of all people, all cultures. We clearly share one life, one earth. We all breathe the same, and we all have families. Yet at the same time, we are wildly different and utterly unique, and we celebrate our interesting, astonishing diversity.

Afterword

In this book, I have intentionally not used the word *Yoga* to describe the Promise Practice. Many readers will have recognized by now that the understandings and application of the Promise are indeed the ancient teachings of Yoga delivered in our modern context. The reason I have chosen not to use the word itself is to offer this practice to the broadest possible public without putting off some readers who may have preconceptions about Yoga, or may have had disappointing experiences attempting to learn or practice it.

Nonetheless, Yoga was the source from which sublime human experience arose. Later this yogic knowledge was converted into abstract meaning through written texts, not only stripping the knowledge of its origins but also imposing the human filter of doctrine and power structure. In this way, the true essence of Yoga was taken from the public. Yoga was distorted and dissociated from its ancient form. Certainly there is much that is sublime in the ancient texts, but its written expression tends to create a desire to strive for their abstract ideals. By *abstract,* I simply mean removed from actual experience, leaving only a description or definition. In fact, though, Yoga *is* the practical means that allows you to experience these ideals directly. You participate in and become intimate with your Nurturing Source Reality through Yoga, but that participation has been lost.

My goal in the Promise is to make available to all people the tools that will make their vision attainable. The Promise embodies our intrinsic union with all ordinary conditions, including the inborn male and female embrace of the natural wonder of life that we share. Yoga is the original means of experiencing God. Even the beautiful idea of the avataric appearance of God on earth in human form (as in the Christian tradition, for example) occurred within the context of Yogic practice. Yoga was the method by which a person could respond and live stably in the presence of such a One, born as the perfect truth that pervades everything.

It is of interest that the ancient texts state that the avatars, often the focus of religious institutions, are paradoxically not the best teachers because they have not been through the process of overcoming personal obstructions to human freedom. Those teachers who have followed the hero's journey to freedom through their own suffering now understand individuals' needs, and they know how Yoga is given appropriately in each situation. I am hoping that all who read this book and take up the Promise Practice will become such teachers, known in the ancient world as *acharya*. In the great tradition, the Avatar and the acharya always worked in a cooperative way in service of one great tradition and purpose. The acharya was needed to show each person how to respond to grace in a real and practical way. Each teaching function was greatly respected. It was said that the qualification to teach had only three aspects.

1. That you had a good teacher yourself;
2. That you practice yourself; and
3. That you care for others.

As I learned from the masters who taught me, the teacher is "no more than a friend and no less than a friend"—not an authority or power structure but a sincere, caring force in local community.

What am I saying here? The usual social model for personal transformation is to form a relationship with the wise person who knows some secrets and methods for you to be free and happy. You listen carefully and try to implement the good ideas. From the ancient masters to the psychiatrist and psychotherapist, every version of this model abounds in the Old World and the new age. We do our darnedest to get it right for ourselves with those elevated figures on the stage, on the pedestal, in the special clothes. We want to emulate them and follow all manner and means to "get there," to what they appear to have: peace, love, bliss; to become freed, centered, balanced, perhaps even become enlightened!

Civilization has been built on this model. But the model implies that you are not there yet; that you are opposite to what you are trying to reach. Throughout the Promise, I have undermined this very assumption because it creates more problems than it solves. It makes our mind and emotions busy with ourselves and our striving, and in the end it leaves us only with a sense of lack. The social model of trying to get there, from the advice of "the man"—the guru or robed figure on stage, male or female, who supposedly knows more than we do—is the very thing that prevents us from enjoying the peace and power of life that is our birthright.

Sorry to say, trying to be like "the man" just does not work. I have seen seekers following their teachers for decades, only to be frustrated that they never seem to "get it." Sometimes the teachers grow disheartened too. But when a teacher can teach actual self-empowerment—each person's unique intimate connection with his or her own life and universe—the teaching comes alive. It is no longer abstract; no longer a search. Trying to be something we are not is the source of our suffering. Buddha and Jesus both knew this and taught the love of mutuality between actual people, although they expressed it in somewhat different terms.

The teacher who will give you the practical tools to enjoy intimate connection to your own life is your friend and true helper. With those tools, you can stop looking and start living your inborn connection to your life by way of body, breath, and all natural relatedness in this vast universe. You stop scurrying to "get there" and start enjoying a life in your own wonder.

The public needs to understand that Yoga is not religion. It is not Hinduism or Taoism and does not belong in any particular camp. Yet it is extremely helpful as the principal tool for religious purposes. It is one of the six *darshanas,* or philosophical systems of the ancient world. The other philosophical systems developed into world religions, while Yoga was and is universal to them all. This is why Yoga flourished everywhere in the ancient world, through all language groups and religious systems, just as it is spreading now through our multicultural contemporary world. It is a necessary part of all faiths and ways of life that are dedicated to improving human life.

Yoga must be given to all people everywhere, just like food and water must be given to all people everywhere. There is a right Yoga for every person, one that takes into account her utter uniqueness. I will say forever that practice is each person's *direct* intimacy with reality itself, which is none other than Nurturing Source, always Given (capital G for Given, or for God!).

My Teachers: The Two Krishnas

I would now like to acknowledge "the two Ks" who served as my personal teachers: Professor T. Krishnamacharya and Uppalari Gopala Krishnamurti, both of whom I had the privilege to be with. Ordinary men, not businessmen, not sagacious "holy men," yet serious about life, these gentlemen were mutual friends with deep respect for each other. They loved each other's sincerity and honesty.

Professor Tirumalai Krishnamacharya, known as the Teacher of the teachers, lived 101 useful years and died in 1989. His scholarship laid down the foundation for

Yoga to enter the modern time, yet, curiously, he has been ignored as the West popularized its Yoga brands. He and U. G. Krishnamurti came from different philosophical positions, yet the professor called U. G. "the greatest living Yogi I have met."

U. G. Krishnamurti, widely known by just the initials of his first names, was a Buddha of our time; a natural man. U. G. was considered by some to be an Avatar, yet he dismissed the whole notion of being spiritual. He would often joke about himself, "I didn't fall off the back of a turnip truck, you know?" The anti-guru: although it was pointed out by followers that the word *guru* spelled backward is "you are U. G.," he would say that U. G. stood for "useless guy." He insisted that the gurus and their glamorous teachings have put humankind on the merry-go-round of self-denial, the denial of the extreme intelligence that is already beauty, blooming fully in your own garden. Any kind of seeking denies this fact.

Even as U. G. eschewed the label of omniscient sage or guru, he taught me one to one in the traditional and most practical ways. He got down on the floor and showed me how Yoga is not manipulation of anything. It is pristine participation in the nurturing force of the universe that knows exactly what it is doing in everyOne's case. It is easy, and anyone can do it.

Some people think of U. G. as a fiery philosopher— "the raging sage"—but he was foremost a Yogi. He lived in a cave with Swami Sivananda Saraswati for seven years in his youth, and was deeply informed of the traditions and personalities of India. He interpreted Krishnamacharya's scholarship with utmost precision and economy. They were friends and modern-day sages, although they would never allow that word to be attributed to them.

U. G. was the teacher who, when I expressed amazement at some of his teachings, used to joke, "Don't tell people I said these things. Tell them *you* said it, and you'll make a lot of money." Think about the level of wisdom of a man who would say that, and mean it. Not mere humility but actively deflecting attention and recognition away from himself after spending his entire life acquiring wisdom. It would be equivalent to a master artist—a Vincent van Gogh or a Mark Rothko—not just leaving a painting unsigned but inviting one of his students to sign his own name and proceed to sell it. We can barely conceive of such an action in the West. In case you think I'm exaggerating, open any of his books to the copyright page, and you will find something like this over his signature: "My teaching, if that is the word you want to use, has no copyright. You are free to reproduce, distribute, interpret, misinterpret, distort, garble, do what you like, even claim authorship, without my consent or the permission of anybody." U. G. would say of money and commerce, "Make money, not for its own sake but to feed the people." The mind-bending quotations I gave as the culmination of the Promise Principles were picked up from U. G., and there are many more.

To my teachers, Yoga was not an attempt to sell anything or to get anywhere. It was a participation in one's life. I represent the collaboration of "the two Krishnas" with my own passion. They made the Promise possible, and I am determined that their collective wisdom reach you.

At the same time, I understand that what these remarkable men had to say could be easily misconstrued. And so I want to acknowledge that what I am teaching is a distillation of that wisdom, designed through years of my own teaching to get through to as many people as possible. Without distorting or losing the essence of what my teachers passed on to me, I am translating their wisdom for contemporary society, in such a way that any person can comprehend, and, more important, use.

I mean this in the most sincere and friendly way. What we are talking about in the Promise is something quite different from what is called Yoga in the West. The principles of our founding grandfather, our source scholar Krishnamacharya, must be put into all the Yoga derivatives that have been made up in both the East and the West. The young Brahmin men who had studied briefly with Krishnamacharya as boys went on to establish aggressive, gymnastic styles without the vital information essential for successful personal practice. These offerings are dislodged from the source teaching, the natural union of feminine with male qualities, inhalation and exhalation, strength that receives, within and without. They then exported these styles in a way that exploited the naïveté of the West. They and their Western derivatives have no direct connection with the wisdom tradition of Yoga, despite the belief that teachers in America have somehow reinvented Yoga and champion it legitimately. Some believe that because women mainly represent the Yoga brands of the West, this is a kind of restoration of the feminine. Yet it's largely the same aggressive gymnastics that have been rebranded. For every sincere practitioner who is attracted to these obsessive Yoga exercising systems, there are many, many more who feel left out or intimidated by their obsessive quality—indeed, most of the population. I have heard many sad stories of folks who, in the belief that Yoga could be helpful to them, have had emotionally and even physically crippling experiences in class, being asked to do things they simply cannot do. Often people are suddenly or progressively injured by the inappropriate gymnastics they attempt to perform.

One man I met recently told of being advised to practice Yoga to help with his chronic low back pain. He would dutifully go to classes and follow the DVDs of famous teachers, striving to imitate the poses they displayed. And yet each time, he would end up reinjuring his back, having to seek relief from chiropractors, physical therapists, and pain medications. When he finally tried the Promise Practice, he did so with some trepidation, fearing another injury. Instead he was soon able to do his Seven-Minute Wonder on a daily basis with no pain or negative repercussions.

The contemporary brands of Yoga are typically offering two kinds of exaggerations: either spiritual gymnastics or physical gymnastics, both attempting to reach some kind of idealized goal. As a part of the Western fitness industry, the styles of Yoga are usually linked to fashion merchandising, which may cause various degrees of body

dysmorphic disorder, a condition in which people become excessively concerned about some perceived defect
in their physical features. Alternatively, Yoga is presented
in the context of religious cultism, as part of an obsessive
seeking for a future state called God or enlightenment.
These two poles have attracted only a small segment of
society. Meanwhile, the broader public is legitimately put
off or even scared of Yoga. Therefore, the very people
who need it for personal and spiritual fulfilment are not
getting it. Yet Yoga is for everybody, not only for those
who already look good in a form-fitting leotard—or who
would like to.

I do not mean to be unkind to anyone or to denigrate
any institution. The changes and distortions to the original teachings of the great Yogis follow a similar pattern
to changes that crept into the teachings and life examples
of all the great spiritual masters. Moses, Buddha, Con-
fucius, Jesus, Muhammad, Lao-tze, and others lived the
full expression of their truth, which was often at radical
odds with prevailing institutions and teachings. After they
died and their followers took charge of the "message,"
however, social prejudices and subtle misunderstandings
began to appear. To take one example, the great masters
generally accepted all classes and social castes, and taught
women as freely as men. This was downright revolution-
ary in the context of their cultures. Once the founders
were gone, the cultural presumptions of their followers
reasserted themselves, and women were often separated,
treated more harshly, and kept from positions of power in
the developing hierarchies. The feminine principle itself

was largely covered over, debased, or marginalized by the men in power.

Although the parallels may not be precise, a similar downgrading of the feminine principle of Yoga has taken place during the process of passing the ancient wisdom from the great masters to their followers. Distortions grew further as the teachings made their passage from the Old World to the New. It's a little like the child's game of telephone, in which a message is whispered from person to person around a room, until the final version bears little resemblance to the initial statement.

This may be inevitable in any transmission process, but it is now all the more imperative to return to the original source and recapture the message in its fullness. I'm sure that all teachers are doing their best with the information they have at hand. Even the Pope, for example, is doing his best with the information he has! But I long for the day when the Pope understands and teaches that obedience to God comes not in the denial of the feminine but in surrender *to* the feminine—the natural human state. Perhaps he will teach Yoga to the congregation and give it this tool. One day.

Some years ago, I had a seemingly humorous dream that reflected my wishes. I was at the German Yoga Conference that coincided with the death of Pope John Paul II (now called Blessed), and the Pope, in my dream, had taken off over Germany on his way to heaven. He looked down on the city of Cologne and saw us all at the conference. From his new disembodied reference point, no longer restricted by dogma or cultural frame, he realized what Yoga actually is, and its vital relevance to religious life. He said delightedly, "Ah, Yoga," and he blessed the gathering on his way.

It was a funny dream from which I woke up startled, and I remembered to tell the story to a few hundred Yogis the next day. I was so surprised when many came to tears hearing the story. Catholicism was their cultural background, yet now they were interested in Yoga. They had not quite resolved the two ways as being relevant to each other, which of course they are. The story of Pope John Paul "getting it" and blessing their "path" resolved something in the air.

Krishnamacharya would always say, "Yoga is not information gathering," a statement that has profound implications. There are no straight lines in nature, yet humanity conceived of the straight line as a way to impose mathematical order on our lives. Regrettably, this imposition has become the primary way we live and perceive. Yoga represents the removal of the imagined necessity of linear information, so that we can relax into what is Given. In the Natural State we see that the world is round, even as we still use straight lines!

Yoga is adaptable to all cultures. We must give Yoga in the language that is familiar and relevant to our audiences—that takes into consideration the unique background of everybody, without imposing a new language or unnecessary ideas. We don't need to migrate to another culture or understand ideas that are not our own. No more "yogaspeak" or spiritual voice tones that inevitably create dualistic grasping for abstract ideals. As a simple example, sometimes even time-honored terminology can get in the way of Yoga transmission. Some people are turned on and others just confused by the Sanskrit names of the poses, or *asanas,* that some teachers like to use. Cleaving to the sentiment of the past and its language is not necessary, although it can be a delightful study if you enjoy it. In most cases I find it more helpful to speak in ordinary language that anybody can understand, as my friends do in this book when communicating their actual experiences. For example, Trish King, who lives in New York City, spontaneously and humorously expressed it well. "I am in a relationship with my breath," she told me. "In fact, we are living together. And, oh yes, we are in a lifelong, committed affair."

I love that!

The same goes for the assumption that Yoga is associated with Hindu deities, and asking students to chant to these deities in the Yoga studios. For some it is beautiful and absolutely true, while for others it is confusing if they have no previous knowledge of Hinduism, and when Christian liturgy or Islamic text, or no text, could perhaps be more relevant to them. We must respect each student for who he or she is. The cultures and mythologies of humanity are vast and rich and all worthy of careful attention and interpretation, including our powerful popular culture as it now unfolds. Please, let's use all culture where it is relevant to the student, while respecting a person's background.

For example, in the great mythologies of the ancient world, we find constant reference to the human yearning for intimate connection. The besotted attraction between male and female deities was the ancient analogy of individuals' journey to unification with the whole universe, to God-union. It reflected the personal, discreet passion of this journey. The coming together of the male and female poles signified victory. In the great Indian epic called the *Ramayana,* Lord Ram yearns for his wife, Sita, who has disappeared for years in the dark, desperate days of that time. Ram's loyal devotee Hanuman is known to be so close to him that he is described as Ram's very breath. In his faithfulness, Hanuman rescues Sita and brings her back to Ram, and the lovers are reunited in eternal bliss. Ram's breath returns Sita to Ram!

The breath will return the feminine aspect to everyone's life, within and without. The feminine has gone missing in our common social life. We are longing for our natural state. The male aspects of strength, acquisition, and control alone are no longer adequate. Strength must receive. We must inhale and exhale. Your breath is your loyal Hanuman who will return Sita to you. Your breath is the catalyst that will allow you to enjoy the tangible intimacy with your love, with your opposite, your better half! And it allows you to feel the Source from which all opposites arrive and return, while you will never dissociate from your love and sex again.

Emmanuel Briand's Story

Emmanuel Briand is an IT entrepreneur and business founder based in San Francisco. After I spoke about my teachers, "the two Krishnas," and their insights into the human obsession for answers outside of ourselves, he addressed the question, if that's the case, of why one should practice at all:

I have seen that humanity's habit of seeking for extraordinary experiences negates the absolute mind-blowing experience of the completely ordinary reality. It's a paradox, but it seems the only way to get to what Yoga calls samadhi, *our intrinsic union, is to engage the deep polar energies of ordinary experience, and not to search for extraordinary awareness or experience. Once you are at peace with this concept, you relax and enjoy your life deeply.*

So why do I practice? Why do I wake up in the morning to go through a sequence of postures and a measurement of my breaths? After struggling with this question, I have come to appreciate that the only reason I practice is for the pure enjoyment of it. Any positive physical or mental benefit comes after the fact. Sometimes many strong emotions surface, including fear and anger, which then burn up and work themselves out without my having to act them out in my life. Sometimes it's a strong, heartfelt sense of peace and happiness. The reason I practice is that I deeply enjoy moving, stretching, and breathing. I love spending some intimate time with my breath, and when I experience the pulse in my fingertips, I feel utterly connected to the first heartbeat that pulsed in the first cell of my life. It's the whole universe in me.

Because of this, I practice without the need for any outcomes. But my practice is somehow affecting all my attitudes, and I feel so well. This was not always so! From regular practice, my capacity to listen seems greater. I am open to receive love from my partner, advice from my friends, discontentment from my kids. Because my anger seems to burn itself out, I feel more compassionate toward others. Why do I attribute this to the practice? And have I been conditioned to create an unnecessary link between my practice and the positive outcomes of my life?

I have concluded that it is a practical gift, the essential offering for all people who need to actualize their dreams, whether they are in spiritual context or in the regular secular world, or both. It powerfully removes obstacles from our inner and outer pathways and locates us in our natural state. Perhaps after some time, the need to practice no longer arises. But the practice makes us feel good, and as a side effect, the body feels strong, and our obstructions to an intimate life are removed. It is hard to deny this.

Mark told me this story about the two Ks. Up to the end of his life, Krishnamacharya was extremely humble. One day U. G. explained that the movements of Yoga that Krishnamacharya was teaching him were in conflict with the innate intelligence and movement of life energy of his natural state. And that was why he was modifying the practice significantly as participation only in what is natural. After first trying to convince U. G. that his method of Yoga was supported by ancient texts, Krishnamacharya later admitted that U. G.'s experience was outside his own understanding. He humbly confessed that he felt he had *realized nothing as a seeker. Krishnamacharya was the most honest of men, and U. G. loved him for that. Throughout these honest exchanges, both men stayed close lifelong friends. U. G. has folded Krishnamacharya's scholarship like silk into his realization of the natural state and produces a clarity for humanity that is unparalleled anywhere in the great traditions. Mark has carried this through with his own unique flavor and realization for all of us.*

How You Can Help

Stand for something or you will fall for anything.
Bloom where you have been planted.

THE MOST PROFOUND WAY TO HELP THE WORLD IS TO help yourself by finding your source of peace and power. You, your family, friends, and whole community are the immediate benefactors of your understanding and practice. Experiment for yourself and promise to practice the Promise for the next forty days. Psychologists tell me that making or changing a habit for the duration of forty days can effect a permanent change. Seven minutes a day times forty amounts to 280 minutes—two feature-length movies, that's all! I always joke that if it was good enough for Jesus to spend forty days in the desert, we can practice too for forty days. I ask you as a friend, not an authority.

Your Seven-Minute Wonder will empower you as an individual and, consequently, the community of which you are a part. We live in a challenging time. This is the worst of times and the best of times. We live in a world where this information is freely available through every media and means of communication everywhere. We are able to develop ways of living that nurture and sustain us amid all the stress in our lives. The practices that are given within these pages are principles that allow you to make your life and practice entirely your own in the great nurturing that lives us all. They will help you truly in the midst of your difficulties. I promise.

As I've said before, there are good teachers in the world, and you may be one of them. They are always ordinary people who care about others, practice, and have good teachers themselves. You do not have to go through enormous amounts of study of difficult practices or traditions. Yoga is not information gathering, and the arbitrary boxes of information that are currently sold as teacher training have little to do with real practice or with the ability to teach. The qualifications to teach are sincerity and the basic knowledge contained here. Such qualified teachers are genuinely concerned for you, and are willing to share information generously. Teaching in this way is not commercial activity but caring for others at a local level. Remember, teachers are no more and no less than friends and are serious about life—and I don't mean humorless! If you are such a person, please teach what you have learned and experienced through your own practice as a friend to as many people who want to learn from you, without forcing it on anybody. This is easier than you might imagine. One of my students was able to teach without language. My friend Bob Dolman reports:

Today I had coffee with Masha Sapron. Masha is a teacher, and recently she was hired by a hotel here in Los Angeles to teach the Promise to hotel employees, because the owner believes that the practice will benefit his workers. So Masha had been leading classes for a while when I met with her. Most of her students are Hispanic and work in housekeeping, cleaning up the hotel rooms. They speak little English, and Masha knows very little Spanish. All Masha says in these classes is inhale and exhale: "Respira profundo, saca el aire."

And it's enough! She guides her students through simple movements, and all she tells them is to breathe. They rest deeply and feel so much better in their stressful lives. She and I talked about this with respect to teaching the Promise in other countries. The idea that a practice available to anyone and everyone is beautiful and provokes peace. So little is needed. Breathe in, breathe out, whoever you are, wherever you live. It connects us all, this basic, natural, necessary action. No bias, no prejudice, no fences. A simple activity from which no one is excluded. Arab, Jew, Protestant, Catholic, Democrat, Republican—we are all unique, yet so connected in this One Life.

Respira profundo. Saca el aire. *Peace is breaking out!*

Give this book to people who will benefit and grow from the practices. The Promise is a healing balm, a warm blanket that can be spread across the world. Go to the websites and interact with the worldwide community. Get the online tutorials, watch the videos, and see how the practice is done. Get involved in the worldwide teaching programs. If we cannot meet face to face, I want to make this message as friendly and personal as possible in every way. Through online communication, much can be shared. May we together offer the Promise to as many as possible all over this suffering world as a means for all of us to enjoy the infinite nurturing force that is life.

On casual observation, it might seem that simply moving and breathing doesn't amount to much. Nonetheless, this practice is more powerful and more fruitful than you would think. So I invite you to try it out for yourself, and practice every day for forty days and see what happens.

Kristi Rugam's Story

I am particularly interested to see how people adapt the Promise to their own background and cultural practices. I was moved by the story of Kristi, a young woman from Estonia whom I met only once. Her simple truth, told not in her mother tongue but in her second or third language, touched a chord. In her case, she was adapting the Promise to a Japanese-based martial arts form called *Shindo*. The Promise adds value and is not necessarily an alternative to a person's lifestyle. She speaks of how the Promise affected her and her teaching in her community:

I am twenty-six years. I am from Estonia and an instructor of Shindo. These Japanese stretches are developed to balance our body and mind, and they work like tools for building the bridges between them. I have led my classes for eighteen months now, and from the first day, I have recognized how important it is to share valuable information. Once you start seeing the world in wider perspective, this commitment comes naturally. I think that we, simple people, are the ones who are creating this world and our surroundings. All that you are is all that there is, nothing more and nothing less! That point gives me the energy and power to share what I have to help others. It does not need a lot, just goodwill that comes from the heart, and we all have it. It is amazing to feel this inside you and spread it out. It goes into life and materializes.

I encourage you to share what you believe and what really counts, whatever has helped you! This is how you can help others. Don't worry, you do not have to influence masses. The right persons eventually will find their way to you. Usually I have only three or four people attending my class at a time. I have such friendly contact with them, and I share my philosophy.

I also do believe that philosophy, which means love of wisdom, is alive, and it transforms and changes with you. Philosophy is organic, and it needs space to live, expand, and stretch out its branches. Don't try to make your philosophy an absolute fact. Believe in it, but don't harass it. Yoga, Shindo, and philosophy—they are free. I see the truth in this point every time I hear something inspiring. I had my great inspiration boost in Bali, where I was discovering and building up my spiritual world. Yes, I can admit, I was searching for it! Not desperately, but I was carried away by the thoughts of meditating with crossed feet, trying to become enlightened and searching all these extreme values outside, not inside, my body! Then I learned the Promise Practice, and I am so grateful. It really helped me to shake off all the pressure from outside and concentrate on who I am, helped me to love myself as I am, and understand what Life (with capital L) has already given to me. I am here now, so I can start living and stop looking for it! Thank you so much, Mark, for sharing!

Later, when I arrived back home in Estonia, I started to see *how it all came together and how my understanding reached deeper. It totally matched with my ideas of Shindo as a simple practice. It was amended by the Promise points that allow actual loving, "in you as you," and seeing the ultimate power. Great finding, isn't it?!*

To sum it up, I want you to know that you can always help! Helping is simple. It allows you to open yourself to the world and understand it. It helps you to create your world and keeps your mind broadened, wide open, and curious for life in general. The changes in life can derive only from you, and when you do your simple routines, you can increase awareness and inner potential. Don't be shy! Share it, help others, and see the growth inside yourself and in the world surrounding you. Help to create the better and diverse world around you and the intelligence of you! Put yourself first! This is the essence that I hash over from time to time with my clients, and I really see the inner smile in their faces as they let go all that force and pressure and accept Life and themselves as they naturally are.

From the one who has stopped searching,
Kristi

And, so, let me be the intervention in your life. Let me move you to practice, and then you take it on. You have to decide, take a stand in your life. That is why we call it the Promise. Once you are practicing, perhaps you will serve as that intervention for others. Take the forty-day test, the free trial, then it will become your own! This is an interwoven promise between us. I promise you these powerful results of intimacy in every way, if you will promise me to practice the Promise.

This *is* the practicum by which you can realize everything that inspires you, whatever that may be. Take this pill, because it works. I want everyOne on the planet to know that he or she is completely loved and cared for. It is time. I want you to help me make sure that all people know they are nurtured. Show them how to do their intimacy with this perfect wonder that we are. As my friend said, "You may say I'm a dreamer, but I'm not the only One."

Take the Next Step
With the Seven-Minute Wonder
Forty-Day Promise

I, _____ (insert name), *promise* to commit to my Seven-Minute Wonder for a minimum of forty days.

Signed: _____ (reader's name)

I, Mark Whitwell, *promise* that you will come to embody the power that lives and breathes you.

Mark J Whitwell

Mark Whitwell

Acknowledgments

I ACKNOWLEDGE THE ENTIRE WISDOM TRADITION OF humanity from which the Promise arose and into which I place it back now as its own practical means, the ancient and present enactment of its ideals. I bow down in gratitude to the vast enterprise of culture in all geographies, ancient and modern, that seeks to understand perfect participation in this Wonder in which we find ourselves. This includes every sincere seeker, saint, sage, and Avatar, known or unnoticed, in Buddhist, Baha'i, Christian, Hindu, Muslim, Jewish, Shinto, Sufi, Taoist, indigenous, shamanic, and all other faiths. To those who have not used doctrine merely as a mechanism of power but as heartfelt enquiry into the Real, I am grateful. And to all who, for their own valid reasons, have finished with spiritual language, but whose hearts are hungry too. Each one of us is doing his or her best to see that we all get home. The Promise is a slight and easy shift for everyOne into union and love. To the whole world I offer this healing power of intimate connection, in the certainty that God is appearing as all ordinary conditions. That the bloom of the flower is as mysterious as its Source, just as God and sex are one.

I thank my friend Uppalari Gopala Krishnamurti, the natural man in the Natural State, the fulfillment of the great tradition, and his scholarly friend Professor Tirumalai Krishnamacharya. Together they gave me the certainty that God is as close as your own breath and sex—that the union we seek has already happened.

I thank the team at Atria for making sure you get this. For Sarah Durand and Judith Curr, who first recognized the Promise and its need to be in the world.

I wish to acknowledge all who offered their sincere voice to these pages, and the many more who told their stories that cannot fit into a single book. I thank my brilliant friends Emmanuel Briand, Dr. Roaslie Chapple, Dr. Shelley Cowden, Bob Dolman, Kate Lamb, and Jane Pike, who through their love and skill nurtured this project and kept their gaze out for us all along the watchtower. It is a worldwide community effort.

I thank you and the millions of people everywhere who are practicing and passing this on.

Experience Your Seven-Minute Wonder in This Series of Videos

With your smart phone, you can access the videos below to view the steps of the Promise Practice. To do so, simply download the free app at gettag.mobi. Then hold your phone's camera a few inches away from the tag and enjoy what comes next. You can also visit www.thepromise.com to watch these videos.

Breathing with the Arms (Sitting)

Breathing with the Arms (Standing)

Inhalation into Chest, Exhalation from Abdominal

Demonstrating Forward Bend

Striding Forward Bend and Back Arch

Forward Bend with Twist

Child Pose and Cat Arch

Reach for the Sky

Legs to the Roof, Arms Overhead

The Bridge

Restoration

A Most Vital Conclusion: Rest

* * *

A complete daily sequence: To complement what you have already learned, you can carry with you a complete sequence and follow it each day on the iPromise smart phone app, Android or Apple devices, available at http://www.thepromise.com/ipromise/. And visit http://www.thepromise.com for seminars and additional resources.

ALSO BY MARK WHITWELL

Yoga of Heart:
The Healing Power of Intimate Connection

Printed in the United States
By Bookmasters